The
30-Day
Diabetes Miracle
COOKBOOK

From the Gourmet Kitchen and Cooking School
at Lifestyle Center of America

The
30-Day
Diabetes Miracle
COOKBOOK

Stop Diabetes with an Easy-to-Follow Plant-Based, Carb-Counting Diet

Bonnie House
Diana Fleming, Ph.D., LDN
Linda Brinegar
Linda Kennedy
and Ian Blake Newman

A PERIGEE BOOK

A PERIGEE BOOK
Published by the Penguin Group
Penguin Group (USA) Inc.
375 Hudson Street, New York, New York 10014, USA
Penguin Group (Canada), 90 Eglinton Avenue East, Suite 700, Toronto, Ontario M4P 2Y3, Canada
(a division of Pearson Penguin Canada Inc.)
Penguin Books Ltd., 80 Strand, London WC2R ORL, England
Penguin Group Ireland, 25 St. Stephen's Green, Dublin 2, Ireland (a division of Penguin Books Ltd.)
Penguin Group (Australia), 250 Camberwell Road, Camberwell, Victoria 3124, Australia
(a division of Pearson Australia Group Pty. Ltd.)
Penguin Books India Pvt. Ltd., 11 Community Centre, Panchsheel Park, New Delhi—110 017, India
Penguin Group (NZ), 67 Apollo Drive, Rosedale, North Shore 0632, New Zealand
(a division of Pearson New Zealand Ltd.)
Penguin Books (South Africa) (Pty.) Ltd., 24 Sturdee Avenue, Rosebank, Johannesburg 2196, South Africa

Penguin Books Ltd., Registered Offices: 80 Strand, London WC2R ORL, England

While the author has made every effort to provide accurate telephone numbers and Internet addresses at the time of publication, neither the publisher nor the author assumes any responsibility for errors, or for changes that occur after publication. Further, the publisher does not have any control over and does not assume any responsibility for author or third-party websites or their content.

First edition: May 2008

Library of Congress Cataloging-in-Publication Data

The 30-day diabetes miracle cookbook : stop diabetes with an easy-to-follow
plant-based, carb-counting diet / Bonnie House . . .[et al.].— 1st ed.
   p. cm.
  Includes index.
  "From the Gourmet Kitchen and Cooking School at Lifestyle Center of America."
  ISBN-13: 978-0-399-53421-8
  1. Diabetes—Diet therapy—Recipes. 2. Vegetarian cookery.
I. Title: Thirty-day diabetes miracle cookbook. II. House, Bonnie
RC662.A14 2008
641.5'6314—dc22   2007050474

PRINTED IN THE UNITED STATES OF AMERICA

10 9 8 7 6 5

PUBLISHER'S NOTE: The recipes contained in this book are to be followed exactly as written. The publisher is not responsible for your specific health or allergy needs that may require medical supervision. The publisher is not responsible for any adverse reactions to the recipes contained in this book.

Neither the publisher nor the author is engaged in rendering professional advice or services to the individual reader. The ideas, procedures, and suggestions contained in this book are not intended as a substitute for consulting with your physician. All matters regarding your health require medical supervision. Neither the author nor the publisher shall be liable or responsible for any loss or damage allegedly arising from any information or suggestion in this book.

Most Perigee books are available at special quantity discounts for bulk purchases for sales promotions, premiums, fund-raising, or educational use. Special books, or book excerpts, can also be created to fit specific needs. For details, write: Special Markets, Penguin Group (USA) Inc., 375 Hudson Street, New York, New York 10014.

This book is dedicated to the 3,000 brave alumni of Lifestyle Center of America, who took a chance on a plant-based diet and a brand-new life. We salute you.

Contents

Acknowledgments

TO THE DEDICATED staff of the LCA Cooking School for contributing to these recipes, and for taking on extra work during the cookbook process: Annie Krajewski, Amelia Lopez, and Aubrey Seiler.

To the Windcrest Restaurant team for their unwavering commitment to excellence, hard work, and contribution to the development of these recipes: Toni Baker, David Greer, Becky Krajewski, Greg Lombard, Karen Meely, Joseph Nally, and Kellie Rushing.

To the project coordinators, taskmasters, word processors, editors, and cheerleaders: Amber Ball, Dan Braun, Kevin Brown, Nickie Busch, Kaya Chong, Susan Jones, Sid Lloyd, and Pam Wegmuller, with special thanks to Siedra Caleb.

To our very patient and consummate photographer, David Smith at Davidography, Chattanooga, Tennessee.

To our "guinea pig" taste-testers, who faithfully loaned us their expert taste buds and judgment in service of helping us fine-tune these great recipes.

To our families, for putting up with missed meals and messy home offices: Tony Brinegar, David Hemmer, Franklin House, and Edward Kennedy.

Introduction

WHAT'S SO SPECIAL ABOUT
THE 30-DAY DIABETES MIRACLE COOKBOOK?

THE LAST 100 years of nutrition research has demonstrated unequivocally the benefits of plant-based foods for optimal human health and longevity. But plant-based foods—think potatoes, rice, and breads—are typically carbohydrate-rich foods. A high-carb diet seems like an oxymoron for those with diabetes. As a result, there are virtually no diabetes cookbooks that are plant-based, and probably none that are high-carb. Yet this cookbook is both. It destroys the myth that a high carb, plant based diet is bad for people with diabetes, and it reminds you that a diet primarily based on animal products is bad for people with diabetes.

How does our diet work? As we described in *The 30-Day Diabetes Miracle*, it works in three main ways:

1. **It avoids all animal products, like meat, milk, eggs, and cheese.** A totally plant-based diet allows us to drastically cut unhealthy saturated fat, and totally eliminate unnecessary dietary cholesterol. All the fats in these recipes come from plants, which are rich in good, healthy, *unsaturated* fatty acids, such as those found in nuts and avocados. Just because there's no meat in our recipes, doesn't mean there isn't enough protein—you'll get plenty of the right kind. Plant-based protein is not concentrated; it's offset by fiber and good carbs, so it's easier for the body to use.

2. **It focuses on the right kind of carbohydrates**—the whole, natural kind, still loaded with fiber and other essential nutrients, unlike stripped-down, processed carbs like those in white flour and sugar. So you'll know how many carbs to eat, our menus and recipes include "Carb Choices," now the preferred method of meal planning for those with diabetes who want to achieve excellent blood-sugar goals. Carb counting

is much easier for people to understand and use than Diabetic Exchange Lists, and research has shown it to be very effective in achieving tight control for people with both type-1 and type-2 diabetes.

3. **It takes in to account the Glycemic Index (GI).** Not all carbs are created equal in terms of their blood-sugar response after eating. Some foods can spike blood sugars fast and high. This cookbook generally focuses on low-glycemic carbs, which help regulate your blood sugar.

The 30-Day Diabetes Miracle Cookbook also keeps track of sodium, calories, fat, and fiber through nutritional analyses provided in each recipe. It's the only cookbook of its kind, and the perfect resource for beginning or maintaining a plant-based diabetic diet.

WHAT'S CARB COUNTING?

DIABETIC MEAL PLANNING with our menus and recipes is based on carb counting, which means you're allotted a certain number of Carb Choices per meal. First a quick word on what carbs are. In general, the total carbohydrates in food equal the sum of the sugar, starch, and fiber. But it's only the *net* carbs that people with diabetes need to worry about. The net carbs include the glucose *available* from sugar and starch during the process of digestion. Glucose from sugar and starch can be absorbed from the digestive tract into the bloodstream, and therefore can raise your blood sugar. While fiber is also a carb, it's *not digestible,* so its glucose is *not available* to you. We determine the amount of net carbohydrate in food by subtracting the grams of fiber from the total grams of carbohydrate. That leaves us with a number, in grams, of net carb, from which we determine how many Carb Choices a food constitutes.

WHAT IS A CARB CHOICE?

SIMPLE: 15 GRAMS *net carbohydrate = 1 Carb Choice.* How much is that? One medium apple or orange, one slice of whole wheat bread, ½ cup of beans, ⅓ cup brown rice, or one whole grain cookie.

HOW MANY CARB CHOICES CAN I EAT?

ON AVERAGE, IF you have type-1 or type-2 diabetes, we'd recommend 3 to 5 Carb Choices for breakfast (45 to 75 grams), 3 to 5 for lunch (45 to 75 grams), and 0 to 3 for supper

(0 to 45 grams). Keeping supper's Carb Choices as low as possible will help with your overnight and morning blood sugars (more on that in the introduction to the Breakfast section). Staying within the range of about 9 to 13 Carb Choices (135 to 195 grams) per day will help you experience the best blood-sugar control, weight loss, and overall resolution of your diabetes problems. We've provided portion-size information for all recipes, so you can even count your dessert portion as part of your carb total for the meal.

WHAT WAS OUR PROCESS FOR DECIDING ON RECIPES?

THERE WERE TWO main goals: nutrition and taste; and one lesser goal: ease of preparation. At Lifestyle Center of America, we've been counseling diabetes patients, cooking them food, and teaching them how to cook it for themselves for more than 10 years. All five authors have been practicing a plant-based lifestyle for a combined total of well over 100 years. So we weren't starting from scratch. But we wanted to make sure all these recipes could pass nutrition-science scrutiny as healthful as they could be for people with diabetes. And we wanted to make sure the average person could find the ingredients and make most of the recipes at home without trouble.

Nutrition

In consultation with our doctors, and in light of several recent landmark studies determining the value of a plant-based diet for diabetes, Dr. Diana Fleming and her nutritional services team determined some basic parameters. In general, each recipe should be:

- **Plant-based.** No meat, milk, cheese, eggs, or other animal products. We believe it's animal proteins and fat that are the cause or major contributor to most, if not all, chronic diseases in the Western world, with obesity and diabetes at the top of that list.
- **Cholesterol-free.** That's covered by no animal products. We get all the cholesterol our bodies need through natural processes, and any extra cholesterol we ingest through our diet is unnecessary and unhealthful.
- **Whole grain heavy.** Low on nutritionally bereft, processed food. Delicious desserts, yes, but no Twinkies here.
- **High-fiber.** Enter the whole grains. Most Americans consume about 12 grams of fiber per day. An official "high-fiber" diet means 16 or more grams of fiber per day. Our diet includes *40 to 50* grams of fiber per day! Fiber makes you feel full, but has no calories, and doesn't affect your blood sugar—*it's a miracle!*
- **Low-glycemic.** To reduce blood-sugar spikes and drops. It's high-glycemic foods such as white flour, white potatoes, cornflakes, white sugar, and certain fruits,

that cause a roller-coaster effect in the blood sugar. After the blood sugar sky-rockets, it plummets, leaving you craving more carbs. Because of the high-fiber content of most of our recipes, and because of the right mix of plant-based fats with the right kinds and amounts of carbs, this diet is dramatically lower-glycemic than traditional diabetic diets. High-fiber, low-glycemic foods account for why, on our diet, most people with diabetes can eat two to three meals per day instead of the six recommended by many plans. Please keep in mind, though, that not *every* individual recipe may be low glycemic *for you*: the Glycemic Index (GI) *will* affect different people in different ways—even at different times of the day. So don't use the GI as your *only* menu planning tool.

■ **Low-calorie.** The guests attending our program consume on average 1,250 to 2,100 calories per day (usually closer to the lower end), but feel satisfied because of the high fiber and low GI. By contrast, most adults consume between 2,000 and 3,000 calories per day, and many consume *a lot* more. So, we've developed our recipes to be much lower in calories than those typically eaten on the Standard American Diet.

■ **Not high-fat.** On average, a guest attending our program will get 25 to 28 percent of their total calories from fat—all good, plant-based fat. Where we have included higher fat favorites such as Classic Hummus (page 217, a traditional Mediterranean bean spread), in almost every case we have also offered a lower fat alternative. Most professional health agencies recommend you eat less than 30 percent of your calories from fat—and they claim it's okay to get most of it from "lean meats" like chicken; we strongly disagree.

■ **Low-saturated fat.** Mainly by eliminating animal products, we've gotten this "unhealthy fat" down to about 4 percent of total calories on average, which is less than one-third of the amount eaten by the average American.

■ **Trans-fat-free.** No partially hydrogenated (or fully hydrogenated) fat typically found in many desserts, snack foods, or processed foods in general. The average American's total caloric intake includes about 2.6 percent trans-fat, which is way too much if you're trying to keep your weight, cholesterol, and heart disease risk down.

■ **Low-sodium.** No more than 550 milligrams per serving, with most recipes much lower per serving. If you're used to salty foods, we urge you to give your taste buds a few weeks to adapt. You'll be surprised.

■ **Proper protein.** On average, for a guest enjoying our total plant-based cuisine, protein accounts for about 15 percent of total calories, a health-protecting level that's not way too high, as it is in the Standard American Diet. Plant-based means you get none of the concentrated protein calories associated with animal products (and no animal diseases, either).

Taste

Next, we considered taste, and here's where we had a lot of honing to do. You need trial-and-error to keep a recipe within those strict nutritional parameters and still make it taste good. We relied on surveys, formal and informal, from a few thousand "guinea pigs" at Windcrest Restaurant in Sulphur, Oklahoma, students at our cooking school, and program alums who've tested recipes at home. Based on these detailed surveys, we culled our recipes down to a group of potential candidates for the book. Then the four principle "cookbook ladies" got together a lot, to cook, taste, refine, and recook. The pictures on the back cover is from one such adventure. For months, there was constant retooling of ingredients, to ensure recipes made the nutritional cut yet still wowed the crowds. Then we went into an exhaustive (and exhausting) "beta-testing" phase, during which we did a lot of cooking and recooking and formally surveyed our staff on all aspects of the recipes. We got great suggestions for revisions from this process, and the LCA staff got stuffed.

Ease of preparation

Finally, we considered how "quick and easy" these recipes would be for the average working person. Are the ingredients, albeit sometimes unfamiliar, accessible in most parts of the country? Do the cooking techniques require a degree in culinary arts? Would you have to mortgage your house to buy the necessary equipment? In judging the ease of preparation, we relied on comments from our former guests who've been making this food at home for years using our recipes. While not every recipe in this book is equally simple and fast—we wanted to include some special-occasion masterpieces—we're confident that no recipe here is beyond the scope of a beginning cook. If you find yourself unfamiliar with a certain ingredient or cooking term, you can find glossaries in the appendices. You can also find information on how to stock your pantry for plant-based cooking, and even a shopping list of brands we endorse. Below is information on one product you'll see a lot of in this cookbook.

WHAT'S THE STORY WITH SOY?

SOYBEANS ARE THE highest quality protein in the plant kingdom—on par with the protein in meat and eggs but minus the bad stuff, the saturated fat and cholesterol, and loaded with the good stuff: fiber, vitamins, minerals, and phytochemicals. Numerous research studies have demonstrated the superior nutritional health benefits of soy. We're impressed with the utility and versatility of soybeans for preparing various meals. Consequently, you'll find a great number of recipes in this cookbook using a range of soy products—from soymilk and tofu to whole beans and ready-made soy products. Following is a brief description of the soy products that we use most often. Our recipes were developed to demonstrate to our LCA guests, most of whom are used to the Standard American Diet, the breadth of possibilities of a plant-based diet. Rest assured this does not mean that we think that you should eat soy or soy products at every meal in order to eat a good plant-based diet. On the contrary, one can eat an excellent plant-based diet without eating soy or tofu, thanks to the vast array of beans throughout the world, most of which also provide superb protein.

Soybeans, whole dried

Soybeans can be cooked and used in sauces, stews, and soups. Store in a dry, airtight container. One cup of dried beans will yield 2½ to 3 cups of cooked beans. Dried soybeans must be thoroughly cooked to be digestible. (When properly cooked, soybeans should be soft enough to easily squish between two fingers.) A pressure cooker is the quickest way to cook soybeans, as the stovetop method will take 2 to 3 hours, even if the soybeans have been presoaked. See Cooking Beans and Legumes (page 10).

Soybeans, green

Usually called edamame, you can buy these beans in or out of their fuzzy green pods. Look for them fresh or frozen in natural-foods stores and well-stocked grocery stores. They keep frozen for several months. Boil in lightly salted water for about 5 minutes. They can be eaten as a serving of excellent quality protein, or added to salads or soups.

Soymilk

It's come a long way since the 1970s when people had to make it from scratch, starting with beans. You can use it in almost any way that dairy milk is used (but be warned: some soymilks do not thicken instant puddings or whip very well). Available whole; low-fat; "lite"; low-carb; flavored (vanilla, almond, cappuccino); and fortified with vitamins B, D, and E, calcium, and beta-carotene. If you're on a strict plant-based diet, we recommend you use a soymilk fortified with vitamin B_{12}. Remember to shake a container of fortified soymilk because the vitamins and minerals tend to settle at the bottom. *Be aware that plain (unflavored), unsweetened soymilk is usually best for cooking.* If you're transitioning from dairy milk and don't immediately adapt to the taste of plain soymilk, add vanilla or a small amount of a natural, low-glycemic sweetener as you transition. Keep soymilk refrigerated after it's opened. You can also buy soymilk powder (store in a dry, sealed container in the refrigerator or freezer), which you can rehydrate with water and use like regular soymilk. Natural-foods stores and nearly all grocery stores now sell soymilk. *Always check the grams of sugar per serving of commercial soymilks or soymilk powders.* Many are loaded with sugar, especially the flavored kinds. We recommend 5 grams of sugar or less per serving.

Tofu

Sometimes called soybean curd, tofu is a soft white food with a cheeselike consistency, made by curdling hot soymilk with a coagulant, then pressing it into a block. Because tofu takes on whatever flavor is added to it, it's a favorite with cooks, and is a staple in Asian cuisine. Tofu is produced in "silken," soft, medium, firm, and extra-firm textures, and in regular, low-fat, or "lite" varieties. Firmer tofus, usually packed in water, are best for slicing, cubing, scrambling, and crumbling into stir-fried, grilled, and baked recipes, as well as soups, when you want the tofu to hold its shape. The softer and silken varieties, usually sold vacuum-sealed, are best for blending, or as a replacement for cream cheese, sour cream, or yogurt in recipes. While about half the calories in regular tofu come from fat, its calorie content is actually quite low. You would have to eat a huge amount to get an appreciable amount of fat (½ pound tofu contains only 10 grams of fat). Tofu is also very low in unhealthy, saturated fat.

Tofu is sold fresh, refrigerated, in bulk, water-packed, or vacuum-packed, as well as in aseptic packaging (the latter requires no refrigeration until opening). You can freeze unused portions of unexpired tofu, wrapped in plastic or foil. It will keep frozen for several months, but its consistency will change to chewy and spongy. After defrosting, carefully squeeze out the water. Look for tofu in supermarkets, either in the produce, dairy, or health foods section. Store your water-packed tofu in the refrigerator, watching the expiration date. Once water-packed tofu is opened, change the water daily. If it turns pink or starts to smell sour, throw it out. You can also buy freeze-dried tofu—great for camping, hiking, or traveling. Reconstitute it in water until it swells. Most of our recipes that contain tofu will keep for 3 days to a week, refrigerated.

Soy sauce

This popular fermented ingredient is used for flavoring, especially in Asian cuisine. We use it in limited quantities because it contains high concentrations of sodium and has limited nutritional value. In general, people with diabetes are more sensitive to sodium than people who don't have diabetes, so we recommend only low-sodium soy sauce. A lower-sodium soy-based flavoring you'll see used in some of our recipes is Bragg Liquid Aminos. It's lower in sodium than regular soy sauce, unfermented, and contains only soybeans and water.

Ready-made soy products

There are a variety of tasty ready-made soy foods on the market today. Just remember that they can be sources of *concentrated* soy protein, which are not the best for your health, and they can be high in sodium, fat, and sugar. Check the labels to see if they fit within your dietary needs. We recommend you use these products as you transition from an animal- to a plant-based diet, as "condiments," or as recipe ingredients in limited quantities. You can purchase these foods at some grocery stores and all health foods stores. They include a wide variety of items like soy burgers, burritos, hot dogs, breakfast links, sausages, bacon, pizza, lasagne, potpie, cheeses, mayonnaise, salad dressings, ice cream, and coffee creamer.

COOKING TIPS FOR A PLANT-BASED DIET

OUR RECIPES CONTAIN a lot of beans and grains, some varieties of which you might not be used to. We've compiled here some details on their preparation.

COOKING GRAINS
(STOVETOP METHOD)

Grain (1 cup dry)	Water (cups)	Minimum Cook Time (minutes)*	Yield (cups)
Barley flakes	3	30	3
Barley groats	3	75	3½
Buckwheat groats	2	15–20	3½
Bulgur wheat	2	15–20	2½
Cornmeal (whole grain)	3	25	3
Cracked wheat	2	25	2
Oats, old-fashioned rolled	2	15	2
Oat groats	3	45–60	3
Quinoa	2	15–20	4
Rice, brown	2½–3	45–60	3
Rice, wild	3	35–60	4
Rye flakes	2	45–60	2

* Cook times will vary depending on your equipment, altitude, the exact variety of grain, and your taste preference.

COOKING GRAINS
(STOVETOP METHOD)

Grain (1 cup dry)	Water (cups)	Minimum Cook Time (minutes)*	Yield (cups)
Spelt berries	3	120	3
Steel-cut oats	3	40–45	3
Whole wheat, cracked	3	45–60	3
Whole wheat berries	3	120	2

*Cook times will vary depending on your equipment, altitude, the exact variety of grain, and your taste preference.

Basic grain cooking directions

Use a covered pan and bring salted water (½ teaspoon per 4 cups water) to a boil. Add the grain while stirring. Return to a boil, lower heat, and simmer for the recommended time. Do not stir whole grains unless you want them creamy and sticky.

Toasting

All grains can be lightly toasted before cooking to enhance flavors and reduce cooking time. Toast in a 250°F oven or a frying pan over low heat until the grain is golden brown. For the frying pan method, place grain in a dry pan (no oil) and constantly stir or turn the grain until golden. Note: Overcooking or blackening the grain risks turning it carcinogenic.

Slow cooker method

Recommended for whole barley, oat groats, and spelt, rye, and wheat berries (you can experiment and mix these, too). Use 4 cups water to 1 cup of grain. Place the grain, hot water, and salt in a slow cooker. Stir briefly to mix. Turn the pot on low and leave overnight (6 to 8 hours).

COOKING BEANS AND LEGUMES
(STOVETOP AND PRESSURE COOKER METHODS)

Bean Type	Soak?*	Stovetop Cook Time (minutes)	Pressure Cooker (minutes)**
Adzuki	Yes	60	5–7
Black (Turtle)	Yes	90	5–8
Black-eyed peas	No	60	Not recommended
Chickpeas (Garbanzo)	Yes	90–150	5–7
Great Northern	Yes	90	5–7
Kidney (red)	Yes	120	5–8
Lentils, brown	No	40–50	Not recommended
Lentils, red	No	25	Not recommended
Lima, large	Yes	90	Not recommended
Navy	No	90	5–7
Peas (small white)	Yes	60–90	5–8
Pinto	Yes	120	5–7
Red	Yes	60–90	6–8
Soybeans	Yes	120–180	12–15
Split peas (green or yellow)	No	45	Not recommended

*When soaking is required, soak the beans overnight (6 to 8 hours), or bring them to a rapid boil, turn off heat, and wait until the beans have plumped, 30 to 60 minutes. Rinse well, place in a pot with half the salt and cover with 2 inches of water. Bring the beans to a boil and cook the specified amount of time. Salt to taste when beans are tender.

**The new, progressive pressure cookers are easy and safe to operate. When using a pressure cooker, follow the manufacturer's instructions. Do not fill your pressure cooker more than half full of beans and liquid, or beyond the recommended line.

Basic bean cooking directions

Cook in salted water (1 teaspoon per 4 cups water) with the lid on.

Slow cooker method

A slow cooker can be used for any bean, but it's especially recommended for longer-cooking ones such as chickpeas and soybeans. Start beans on the stove and heat to the boiling point, or start beans on the high setting for 2 hours. Then set on low and cook overnight (6 to 8 hours) with 3 inches of water, broth, or stock covering the beans. Add salt, if desired, at the end of cooking.

BEAN AND LEGUME NOTES

1. Always wash beans and legumes thoroughly. Sometimes the packages contain soil, small stones, or other debris. Make sure your beans are fresh. Old beans take longer to cook—if they cook at all.
2. Beans and legumes must be completely cooked to destroy harmful toxins and render them easily digestible.
3. We tested all the cooking times given in the tables using standard equipment, but nothing is exact in cooking. Cooking times may vary according to your equipment, the exact variety and age of the beans, even your altitude.

BEANS, BEANS, THE MUSICAL FRUIT . . .

THERE ARE A few techniques you can use to avoid or reduce the gas and bloating problem associated with increasing your bean intake.

How to cook beans to reduce gas method #1

1. If soaking is required, soak overnight (6 to 8 hours). Do not save the water.
2. Rinse the beans very well.
3. Add fresh water, bring the beans to a boil, then simmer uncovered for 3 to 5 minutes.
4. Cool, then wash the beans once more before cooking for the time specified.

How to cook beans to reduce gas method #2

1. For beans that don't require soaking, bring the beans and water to a boil and let set until the beans are plumped, about 1 hour. Strain the beans and add fresh water.
2. Put the parboiled beans into a slow cooker, pressure cooker, or on the stovetop and cook until tender.
3. Cook on low overnight (6 to 8 hours) if using a slow cooker.

How to eat beans to reduce gas

1. Chew beans (and all plant-based foods) very thoroughly. When larger chunks of vegetable matter reach the intestinal tract, bacteria there have more to work on, which produces excess gas. If you chew thoroughly, though, digestive enzymes and saliva begin to break down the vegetable matter, and less gas will be produced later.

2. Drink lots of water between meals when you're on a plant-based diet high in beans. This will move food more quickly through your digestive tract.

3. If possible, eat foods that are a little harder to digest (like beans) at the beginning of your meal, and follow with foods that are easier to digest, like grains.

4. If you find you have a gas problem, try not combining fruits and beans. Sugars from fruit, especially melons, ferment and mix with carbs from beans that we don't digest well, but our gas-producing bacteria do.

5. Eat smaller meals in general.

6. Be patient: Occurrences of gas decrease through adaptability after a few weeks or months.

CONVERTING UNHEALTHFUL TRADITIONAL RECIPES TO PLANT-BASED TREATS

WHILE ALL OF our recipes are totally plant-based, you might encounter some of your own favorite "traditional" recipes that you want to convert to plant-based recipes for health reasons. Here are some pointers:

PLANT-BASED SUBSTITUTIONS

Animal Product	Plant-Based Substitution
1 cup cow's milk	1 cup fortified soymilk, grain (e.g., rice) milk, or nut milk *Note: Soymilk doesn't whip well in puddings.*
1 cup buttermilk	1 cup soymilk plus 2 teaspoons lemon juice
1 cup cottage cheese	1 cup mashed, water-packed tofu, drained and seasoned
½ cup cream cheese	½ cup soy cream cheese
1 egg *Note: See details on plant-based egg substitutes below.*	• 1 tablespoon ground flaxseed mixed with 3 tablespoons water • 2–4 tablespoons soft tofu • ¼ cup mashed very ripe banana or applesauce • ¼ cup soy yogurt • 1 teaspoon Ener-G Egg Replacer for baking • 1½ teaspoons Ener-G Egg Replacer plus 2 tablespoons water, whisked well. *Use as a binder only in casseroles, cookies, nut balls, etc. Leaves some items, like cookies, crispy.*

Animal Product	Plant-Based Substitution
1 serving meat	• Equal amounts of soy or gluten substitute • Beans • Tofu • Tempeh • Portobello mushrooms
1 cup meat or chicken stock	• 1 cup liquid vegetable stock • 1 cup water plus vegetable stock cubes or powder • 1 cup water plus Bragg Liquid Aminos or low-sodium soy sauce, to taste
1 cup white sugar	1 cup dried cane juice crystals or fructose

PLANT-BASED EGG SUBSTITUTES

1. **Flaxseed.** Works best in whole grain recipes such as pancakes, muffins, cookies, and some cakes. Flax has a whole grain taste, so put it in recipes where its flavor will blend well. Finely grind the flax in a coffee grinder. Add water and whisk until gooey and gelatinous, much like an egg white. Pre-ground flax has to be kept in the refrigerator or freezer.
2. **Silken Tofu Recipe #1.** Works best in dense cakes, brownies, and cornbread. If the recipe calls for 3 eggs, use only 2 "tofu" eggs (¼ cup silken tofu = 1 egg). Whiz in a blender with other wet ingredients until completely smooth and creamy.
3. **Silken Tofu Recipe #2.** Works best in lighter cakes and muffins. Can make some recipes, such as cookies, seem too cakelike. Blend 1 (12.3-ounce) carton Mori-Nu lite, firm silken tofu with 1 cup water and 2 tablespoons lemon juice until smooth and creamy. Yield is 2½ cups (¼ cup = 1 egg white).*
4. **Soy Yogurt.** Works best in quick breads, muffins, and cakes (¼ cup soy yogurt = 1 egg). Yogurt works a lot like blended tofu. It makes things moist, so use in whole grain recipes.

* Source: *Great Good Desserts Naturally,* by Fran Costigan (Good Cakes Publications, 2000).

Following is a month's worth of menus, complete with portion sizes and Carb Choices. Daily Carb Choices range from 9 to 10. To get the full effect of the "miracle," we encourage readers with diabetes to follow these menus (you can mix and match as long as you stick within the daily range of 9 to 10 Carb Choices), and to watch portion sizes.

Sunday

MEAL	PORTION SIZE	CARB CHOICES (number)
Breakfast		
Golden Soy Oat Pancakes (page 58)	3 pancakes	1½
Very Berry Topping (page 77)	⅔ cup	1
Breakfast Great Northern Beans (page 51)	½ cup	1
Almonds	½ ounce (11–12 nuts)	free
Milk/unsweetened soy or almond	½ cup	free
Ground Flaxseed (page 64)	1–2 tablespoons	free
Lunch		
Black Bean Enchilada (page 132)	1 enchilada	1½
Rustic Quinoa Pilaf (page 197)	¾ cup	1½
Steamed broccoli	1½ cups	free
Garden salad	2 cups	free
Creamy Ranch Dressing (page 104)	2 tablespoons	free
Key Lime Pie à la Linda B. (page 254)	1/16 pie	1
Dinner		
Chickpea Noodle Soup (page 83)	1 cup	1⅓
Caesar Salad (page 101)	2 cups	½
Total Carb Choices		9⅓

Monday

MEAL	PORTION SIZE	CARB CHOICES (number)
Breakfast		
7-Grain Cereal Plus (page 47)	1 cup	1⅓
Breakfast Pinto Beans (page 52)	½ cup	1
Ezekiel 4:9 Sprouted Grain bread	1 slice, toasted	1
Almond butter	1 tablespoon	free
Apple	1 medium	1
Milk/unsweetened soy or almond	½ cup	free
Ground Flaxseed (page 64)	1–2 tablespoons	free
Lunch		
Deluxe Lentil Soup (page 135)	1 cup	1
Sunburst Salad (page 115)	2 cups	1
Steamed fresh zucchini	1 cup	free
Southern Country Cornbread (page 180)	2-inch square	1
Blueberries	½ cup	½
Dinner		
Cream of Asparagus Soup (page 84)	1 cup	1
Garden salad	2 cups	free
LCA Low-Sodium House Dressing (page 110)	2 tablespoons	free
Total Carb Choices		9

Tuesday

MEAL	PORTION SIZE	CARB CHOICES (number)
Breakfast		
Traditional Scrambled Tofu (page 75)	1 cup	½
Ezekiel 4:9 Sprouted Grain bread	1 slice, toasted	1
Smart Balance Light Buttery Spread	2 teaspoons	free
Pear	1 medium	1⅓
Pecans	½ ounce (10 halves)	free
Ground Flaxseed (page 64)	1–2 tablespoons	free
Lunch		
Whole grain pasta with	1 cup	2
Nut Meatballs (page 148)	4 balls	⅔
Chunky Marinara Sauce (page 216)	¾ cup	½
Sugar snap peas	1 cup	½
Strawberry-Spinach Salad (page 114)	2 cups	⅔
Dinner		
Spicy Vegetable Quinoa Soup (page 95)	1 cup	1⅓
Garden salad	2 cups	free
LCA Low-Sodium House Dressing (page 110)	2 tablespoons	free
Apple	1 medium	1
Total Carb Choices		9½

Wednesday

MEAL	PORTION SIZE	CARB CHOICES (number)
Breakfast		
Great Groats and Oats (page 67)	1 cup	2
Kickin' Western Chili (page 143)	1 cup	1⅓
Strawberries	1 cup	½
Walnuts	½ ounce (7 halves)	free
Milk/unsweetened soy or almond	½ cup	free
Ground Flaxseed (page 64)	1–2 tablespoons	free
Lunch		
Tofu Egg Salad Pita		
Tofu Egg Salad (page 234)	½ cup per ½ pita	⅔
Ezekiel 4:9 Prophet's pocket bread	2 half pita pockets	1
Lettuce leaves, tomato slices, and red onion rings in each half pocket		free
Raw vegetables: broccoli, cauliflower, cucumbers, baby carrots, or peppers	1½ cups	free
Creamy Ranch Dressing (page 104) for dipping	¼ cup	free
Peanut Butter–Flaxseed Cookies (page 260)	1 cookie	1
Dinner		
Mediterranean Barley and Lentil Soup (page 90)	1 cup	1½
Ezekiel 4:9 Sprouted Grain bread	1 slice, toasted	1
Smart Balance Light Buttery Spread	2 teaspoons	free
Total Carb Choices		9

Thursday

MEAL	PORTION SIZE	CARB CHOICES (number)
Breakfast		
Alpine Muesli (page 48)	1⅔ cups	3½
Grapefruit	1	1
Lunch		
Linda B.'s Sesame Lettuce Wraps (page 146)	1 wrap	½
Thai Peanut Sauce (page 232)	1 tablespoon	free
Stir-Fried Vegetables (page 202)	1½ cups	1
Mellow Brown Rice (page 194)	⅓ cup	1
Edamame (page 187)	½ cup	⅔
Garden salad	2 cups	free
Annie's Gingery Vinaigrette	2 tablespoons	free
Dinner		
Garden Minestrone Soup (page 87)	1 cup	⅔
Ryvita dark rye crackers	2 crackers	1
Garden salad	2 cups	free
Fat-Free Italian Dressing (page 108)	2 tablespoons	free
Total Carb Choices		9⅓

Friday

MEAL	PORTION SIZE	CARB CHOICES (number)
Breakfast		
Old-Fashioned Rolled Oats (page 70)	1 cup	1½
Breakfast Black Beans (page 50)	½ cup	1
Blueberries	1 cup	1
Almonds	½ ounce (11–12 nuts)	free
Milk/unsweetened soy or almond milk	½ cup	free
Ground Flaxseed (page 64)	1 to 2 tablespoons	free
Lunch		
Haystacks		3 per haystack
Baked tortilla chips	1½ ounces (27 chips)	
Kickin' Western Chili (page 143)	1 cup	
Lettuce, tomato, onion, avocado, black olives, and salsa		
Peach	1 medium	1
Dinner		
Our Favorite Split-Pea Soup (page 91)	2 cups	2
Garden salad	2 cups	free
LCA Low-Sodium House Dressing (page 110)	2 tablespoons	free
Total Carb Choices		9½

Saturday

MEAL	PORTION SIZE	CARB CHOICES (number)
Breakfast		
Chipped Tofu on a Shingle (page 54)	1 cup	1½
Ezekiel 4:9 Sprouted Grain bread	1½ slices, toasted	1½
Breakfast Pinto Beans (page 52)	½ cup	1
Grapefruit	½	½
Brazil nuts	½ ounce (3 nuts)	free
Ground Flaxseed (page 64)	1–2 tablespoons	free
Lunch		
Spinach Lasagne (page 159)	¹⁄₁₆ of 13 × 9-inch pan	1⅓
Steamed baby carrots	1 cup	⅔
Steamed broccoli	1½ cups	free
Caesar Salad (page 101)	2 cups	½
Easy Fruit Salad (page 246)	1½ cups	1
Dinner		
Summer Vegetable Soup (page 96)	2 cups	1
Garden salad	2 cups	free
Creamy Ranch Dressing (page 104)	2 tablespoons	free
Total Carb Choices		9

Sunday

MEAL	PORTION SIZE	CARB CHOICES (number)
Breakfast		
Santa Fe Waffles (page 61)	2 (6-inch) waffles	2⅓
Pico Fresca (page 62)	1 cup	⅓
Banana, green on ends	½ of a 6-inch banana	1
Ground Flaxseed (page 64)	1–2 tablespoons	free
Lunch		
Lemon-Basil Kabobs (page 144)	2 kabobs	1⅓
Ebony Wild Rice (page 193)	⅓ cup	1
Saucy Red Kidney Beans (page 188)	½ cup	1
Steamed broccoli	1½ cups	free
Garden salad	1 cup	free
LCA Low-Sodium House Dressing (page 110)	2 tablespoons	free
Just Plain Good Coconut Cream Pie (page 253)	1/16 pie	1
Dinner		
White Bean and Kale Soup (page 97)	1 cup	1
Garden salad	2 cups	free
Fat-Free Italian Dressing (page 108)	2 tablespoons	free
Total Carb Choices		9

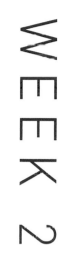

WEEK 2

Monday

MEAL	PORTION SIZE	CARB CHOICES (number)
Breakfast		
Walnut Wheat Berries (page 72)	1 cup	2
Breakfast Great Northern Beans (page 51)	½ cup	1
Peach	1 medium	1
Milk/unsweetened soy or almond	½ cup	free
Ground Flaxseed (page 64)	1–2 tablespoons	free
Lunch		
10-Minute Burger (page 125)		2½ with fixings
veggie burger patty		
Ezekiel 4:9 Sprouted Grain burger bun		
Green leaf lettuce, sliced tomato, and red onion rings		
Low-Fat Tofu Mayonnaise (page 223)	2 tablespoons	free
Sweet Potato Fries (page 203)	1 cup	2
Celery sticks	1 cup	free
Dinner		
Roasted Red Bell Pepper Bisque (page 92)	1 cup	1
Garden salad	2 cups	free
No-Oil Raspberry Dressing (page 111)	2 tablespoons	free
Total Carb Choices		9½

Tuesday

MEAL	PORTION SIZE	CARB CHOICES (number)
Breakfast		
Kashi Go Lean High Protein and High Fiber Cereal	1½ cups	2
Blackberries	1 cup	⅔
100% Sprouted Grain English muffins	½ muffin, toasted	1
Peanut butter, unsweetened, nonhydrogenated	1 tablespoon	free
Milk/unsweetened soy or almond	1 cup	⅓
Ground Flaxseed (page 64)	1–2 tablespoons	free
Lunch		
Sombrero Olé (page 158)		
Ezekiel 4:9 Sprouted Grain tortilla	1	1
Refried Pinto Beans (page 190)	1 cup	2
Lettuce, tomato, onion		free
Guacamole Rico (page 219)	¼ cup	free
Salsa Fresca (page 229)	½ cup	⅓
Pimiento Cheese Sauce (page 228)	2 tablespoons	free
Apple	1 medium	1
Dinner		
Cream of Celery Soup (page 85)	1 cup	1
Garden salad	2 cups	free
Fat-Free Italian Dressing (page 108)	2 tablespoons	free
Total Carb Choices		9⅓

Wednesday

MEAL	PORTION SIZE	CARB CHOICES (number)
Breakfast		
Double Oats (page 66)	1½ cups	3
Breakfast Black Beans (page 50)	½ cup	1
Sweet cherries	1 cup	1
Walnuts	½ ounce (7 halves)	free
Milk/unsweetened soy or almond	½ cup	free
Ground Flaxseed (page 64)	1–2 tablespoons	free
Lunch		
Three Sisters' Stew (page 163)	1 cup	1⅓
Confetti Cornbread (page 181)	2-inch square	1
Steamed broccoli	1½ cups	free
Garden salad	2 cups	free
LCA Low-Sodium House Dressing (page 110)	2 tablespoons	free
Plums	2	1
Dinner		
Down-Home Green Pea Soup (page 86)	1 cup	1
Garden salad	2 cups	free
Creamy Ranch Dressing (page 104)	2 tablespoons	free
Total Carb Choices		9⅓

Thursday

MEAL	PORTION SIZE	CARB CHOICES (number)
Breakfast		
Whole Grain Corn Grits (page 73)	1 cup	2
Pimiento Cheese Sauce (page 228)	2 tablespoons	free
Kickin' Western Chili (page 143)	1 cup	1⅓
Blueberries	1 cup	1
Pecans	½ ounce (10 halves)	free
Ground Flaxseed (page 64)	1–2 tablespoons	free
Lunch		
Tuscan Stuffed Peppers (page 166)	2 halves	1
Seasoned Garbanzos (page 184)	¾ cup	1⅔
Green beans	1 cup	⅓
Garden salad	2 cups	free
Fat-Free Italian Dressing (page 108)	2 tablespoons	free
Dinner		
Southwest Soup (page 94)	1 cup	⅔
Tortilla Strips (page 205)	12 strips	Free
Nectarine	1 medium	1
Total Carb Choices		9

W E E K 2

Friday

MEAL	PORTION SIZE	CARB CHOICES (number)
Breakfast		
Old-Fashioned Rolled Oats (page 70)	1 cup	1½
Breakfast Pinto Beans (page 52)	½ cup	1
Raspberries	1 cup	⅓
Walnuts	½ ounce (7 halves)	free
Milk/unsweetened soy or almond	½ cup	free
Ground Flaxseed (page 64)	1–2 tablespoons	free
Lunch		
Chunky Chickpea Pita Pocket		2½ per sandwich
Chunky Chickpea Spread (page 215)	⅓ cup per ½ pita	
Ezekiel 4:9 Prophet's pocket bread	2 half-pita pockets	
Shredded lettuce and diced tomato		
Cauliflower-Broccoli Salad (page 103)	1 cup	⅔
Diana's Delicious Un-Chocolate Brownies (page 261)	2-inch square	1⅓
Dinner		
Butternut–Black Bean Soup (page 81)	2 cups	2
Garden salad	2 cups	free
LCA Low-Sodium House Dressing (page 110)	2 tablespoons	free
Total Carb Choices		9⅓

Saturday

MEAL	PORTION SIZE	CARB CHOICES (number)
Breakfast		
Cashew Burger Gravy (page 53)	⅔ cup	⅔
Country Barley Biscuits (page 55)	1½ (2-inch) biscuits	1½
Abuela Amelia's Beans (page 175)	1 cup	2
Kiwifruit	2 medium	1
Almonds	½ ounce (11 to 12)	free
Ground Flaxseed (page 64)	1–2 tablespoons	free
Lunch		
Gourmet Eggplant Stacks (page 136)	1 stack	1
Summer squash	1 cup	free
Asparagus	1 cup	free
Saucy Red Kidney Beans (page 188)	¾ cup	1
Garden salad	2 cups	free
Wishbone Olive Oil Vinaigrette	2 tablespoons	free
Apple	1 medium	1
Dinner		
Indian Lentil Soup (page 89)	1 cup	1
Garden salad	2 cups	free
Creamy Ranch Dressing (page 104)	2 tablespoons	free
Total Carb Choices		9⅙

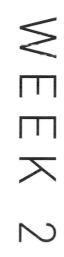

WEEK 2

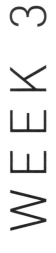

WEEK 3

Sunday

MEAL	PORTION SIZE	CARB CHOICES (number)
Breakfast		
Golden Soy Oat Waffles (page 59)	1 (6-inch) waffle	1⅓
Very Berry Topping (page 77)	1 cup	1⅔
Breakfast Black Beans (page 50)	½ cup	1
Walnuts	½ ounce (7 halves)	free
Milk/unsweetened soy or almond	½ cup	free
Ground Flaxseed (page 64)	1–2 tablespoons	free
Lunch		
Haystacks		3 per haystack
Baked tortilla chips	1½ ounces (27 chips)	
Kickin' Western Chili (page 143)	1 cup	
Lettuce, tomato, onion, avocado, black olives, and salsa		
Pear	1 medium	1⅓
Dinner		
Sautéed Button Mushroom Soup (page 93)	1 cup	⅔
Garden salad	2 cups	free
Fat-Free Italian Dressing (page 108)	2 tablespoons	free
Total Carb Choices		9

Monday

MEAL	PORTION SIZE	CARB CHOICES (number)
Breakfast		
Simply Steel-Cut Oats (page 71)	1 cup	2
Breakfast Great Northern Beans (page 51)	¾ cup	2
Raspberries	1 cup	⅓
Pecans	½ ounce (10 halves)	free
Milk/unsweetened soy or almond	½ cup	free
Ground Flaxseed (page 64)	1–2 tablespoons	free
Lunch		
Kickin' Western Chili (page 143)	1 cup	1⅓
Southern Country Cornbread (page 180)	2 (2-inch) squares	2
Smart Balance Light Buttery Spread	2 teaspoons	free
Garden salad	2 cups	free
LCA Low-Sodium House Dressing (page 110)	2 tablespoons	free
Fancy Fruit Salad (page 247)	½ cup	⅔
Dinner		
Chickpea Noodle Soup (page 83)	1 cup	1⅓
Garden salad	2 cups	free
LCA Low-Sodium House Dressing (page 110)	2 tablespoons	free
	Total Carb Choices	9⅔

WEEK 3

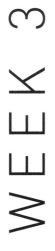

WEEK 3

Tuesday

MEAL	PORTION SIZE	CARB CHOICES (number)
Breakfast		
Creamy Cranberry Quinoa (page 65)	1 cup	2
Kickin' Western Chili (page 143)	¾ cup	1
Sweet cherries	½ cup	½
Walnuts	½ ounce (7 halves)	free
Milk/unsweetened soy or almond	½ cup	free
Ground Flaxseed (page 64)	1–2 tablespoons	free
Lunch		
Alfredo Sauce and Sautéed Mushrooms over Zucchini Ribbons (page 126)	1 serving	⅔
Baked Sweet Potato (page 176)	½ medium	⅔
Tasty Black-Eyed Peas (page 192)	¾ cup	1½
Garden salad	1½ cups	free
No-Oil Raspberry Dressing (page 111)	2 tablespoons	free
Raspberry Swirl Cheesecake (page 268)	1/16 cake	1
Dinner		
Our Favorite Split-Pea Soup (page 91)	2 cups	2
Garden salad	2 cups	free
Creamy Ranch Dressing (page 104)	2 tablespoons	free
Total Carb Choices		9⅓

Wednesday

MEAL	PORTION SIZE	CARB CHOICES (number)
Breakfast		
7-Grain Cereal Plus (page 47)	1 cup	1⅓
Breakfast Pinto Beans (page 52)	½ cup	1
Ezekiel 4:9 Sprouted Grain bread	1 slice, toasted	1
Almond butter	1 tablespoon	free
Orange	1 medium	1
Milk/unsweetened soy or almond	½ cup	free
Ground Flaxseed (page 64)	1–2 tablespoons	free
Lunch		
Baked Falafels (page 129)	2 balls	1
Ezekiel 4:9 Prophet's pocket bread	½ pita pocket	½
Shredded lettuce, diced tomatoes		free
Garlic Tahini Sauce (page 218)	1 tablespoon	free
Smoky Lentils with Caramelized Onions (page 191)	1 cup	2
Tabouli Salad (page 116)	¾ cup	⅔
Dinner		
Garden Minestrone Soup (page 87)	1 cup	⅔
Garden salad	2 cups	free
Fat-Free Italian Dressing (page 108)	2 tablespoons	free
Total Carb Choices		9⅙

WEEK 3

Thursday

MEAL	PORTION SIZE	CARB CHOICES (number)
Breakfast		
Hearty Barley Flakes (page 68)	1 cup	2
Breakfast Black Beans (page 50)	½ cup	1
Blueberries	1 cup	1
Brazil nuts	½ ounce (3 nuts)	free
Milk/unsweetened soy or almond	½ cup	free
Ground Flaxseed (page 64)	1–2 tablespoons	free
Lunch		
Tex-Mex Casserole (page 161)	⅟₁₆ of 13 × 9-inch pan	1½
Guacamole Rico (page 219)	¼ cup	free
Salsa Fresca (page 229)	½ cup	⅓
Yellow squash	1 cup	free
Brilliant Kale with Red Pepper and Onion (page 177)	1 cup	1
Garden salad	2 cups	free
LCA Low-Sodium House Dressing (page 110)	2 tablespoons	free
Dinner		
Mediterranean Barley and Lentil Soup (page 90)	1 cup	1½
Peach	1 medium	1
Total Carb Choices		9⅓

Friday

MEAL	PORTION SIZE	CARB CHOICES (number)
Breakfast		
Great Groats and Oats (page 67)	1 cup	2
Kickin' Western Chili (page 143)	1 cup	1⅓
Strawberries	1 cup	½
Walnuts	½ ounce (7 halves)	free
Milk/unsweetened soy or almond	½ cup	free
Ground Flaxseed (page 64)	1–2 tablespoons	free
Lunch		
Pita Pizza with Low-Fat Lifestyle Hummus (page 154)	1 pizza	2
Steamed broccoli	1½ cups	free
Baked Sweet Potato (page 176)	½ medium	⅔
Garden salad	2 cups	free
Fat-Free Italian Dressing (page 108)	2 tablespoons	free
Fresh Fruit Sorbet (page 248)	⅓ cup	⅔
Dinner		
Cream of Celery Soup (page 85)	1 cup	1
Garden salad	2 cups	free
LCA Low-Sodium House Dressing (page 110)	2 tablespoons	free
Ryvita dark rye crackers	2 crackers	1
Total Carb Choices		9⅙

WEEK 3

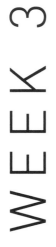

WEEK 3

Saturday

MEAL	PORTION SIZE	CARB CHOICES (number)
Breakfast		
Baked Apple Oats (page 49)	2 servings	2
Abuela Amelia's Beans (page 175)	½ cup	1
Ezekiel 4:9 Sprouted Grain bread	1 slice, toasted	1
Smart Balance Light Buttery Spread	2 teaspoons	free
Blackberries	½ cup	⅓
Milk/unsweetened soy or almond	½ cup	free
Ground Flaxseed (page 64)	1–2 tablespoons	free
Lunch		
Tofoo Yung (page 165)	2 patties	⅓
Two-Color Rice Combo (page 195)	⅔ cup	2
Stir-Fried Vegetables (page 202)	1½ cups	1
Garden salad	2 cups	free
Creamy Ranch Dressing (page 104)	2 tablespoons	free
Apple	1 medium	1
Dinner		
Spicy Vegetable Quinoa Soup (page 95)	1 cup	1⅓
Garden salad	2 cups	free
LCA Low-Sodium House Dressing (page 110)	2 tablespoons	free
Total Carb Choices		10

Sunday

MEAL	PORTION SIZE	CARB CHOICES (number)
Breakfast		
Flaxseed French Toast (page 57)	2 slices	2
Very Berry Topping (page 77)	⅔ cup	1
Breakfast Great Northern Beans (page 51)	½ cup	1
Almonds	½ ounce (11 to 12 nuts)	free
Ground Flaxseed (page 64)	1–2 tablespoons	free
Lunch		
Italian Stuffed Shells (page 141)	2 stuffed shells	1⅓
Seasoned Garbanzos (page 184)	¾ cup	1½
Steamed broccoli	1½ cups	free
Caesar Salad (page 101)	2 cups	½
Classic Lemon Pie (page 251)	¹⁄₁₆ pie	1⅓
Dinner		
Gazpacho (page 88)	1 cup	½
Baked tortilla chips	½ ounce (9 chips)	⅔
Total Carb Choices		10

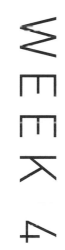

WEEK 4

Monday

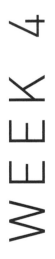

WEEK 4

MEAL	PORTION SIZE	CARB CHOICES (number)
Breakfast		
Oat Bran Cereal (page 69)	1½ cups	1½
Breakfast Pinto Beans (page 52)	¾ cup	1½
Raspberries	1 cup	⅓
Pecans	½ ounce (7 halves)	free
Milk/unsweetened soy or almond	½ cup	free
Ground Flaxseed (page 64)	1–2 tablespoons	free
Lunch		
Grilled Portobello Mushroom Sandwich		
Grilled Portobello Mushrooms (page 138)	1	⅓
Ezekiel 4:9 Sprouted Grain burger bun	1 bun	2
Lettuce leaves, tomato slice, and red onion rings		free
Nayonaise spread	1 tablespoon	free
Sweet Potato Fries (page 203)	1 cup	2
Zippy Kale Salad (page 121)	1½ cups	⅓
Dinner		
Roasted Red Bell Pepper Bisque (page 92)	1 cup	1
Garden salad	2 cups	free
Fat-Free Italian Dressing (page 108)	2 tablespoons	free
Total Carb Choices		9

Tuesday

MEAL	PORTION SIZE	CARB CHOICES (number)
Breakfast		
Whole Grain Corn Grits (page 73)	1 cup	2
Pimiento Cheese Sauce (page 228)	2 tablespoons	free
Abuela Amelia's Beans (page 175)	½ cup	1
Kiwifruit	2 medium	1
Walnuts	½ ounce (7 halves)	free
Ground Flaxseed (page 64)	1–2 tablespoons	free
Lunch		
Grilled Quesadilla (page 139)	1 quesadilla	3
Salsa Fresca (page 229)	2 tablespoons	free
Garden salad	2 cups	free
LCA Low-Sodium House Dressing (page 110)	2 tablespoons	free
Pear	1 medium	1⅓
Dinner		
Butternut Harvest Soup (page 82)	2 cups	1⅓
Garden salad	2 cups	free
No-Oil Raspberry Dressing (page 111)	2 tablespoons	free
Total Carb Choices		9⅔

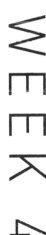

WEEK 4

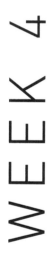

WEEK 4

Wednesday

MEAL	PORTION SIZE	CARB CHOICES (number)
Breakfast		
All Bran—Original	1 cup	1⅔
Kickin' Western Chili (page 143)	¾ cup	1
Blueberries	1 cup	1
Brazil nuts	½ ounce (3 nuts)	free
Milk/unsweetened soy or almond	1 cup	⅓
Ground Flaxseed (page 64)	1–2 tablespoons	free
Lunch		
Succulent Ratatouille (page 160)	1 cup	⅔
Polenta Squares (page 196)	2 squares	1⅓
Sautéed Spinach (page 200)	1 cup	free
Steamed cauliflower	1 cup	free
Green Soybean Salad (page 109)	½ cup	1
Dinner		
Indian Lentil Soup (page 89)	1 cup	1
Garden salad	2 cups	free
Creamy Ranch Dressing (page 104)	2 tablespoons	free
Nectarine	1 medium	1
Total Carb Choices		9

Thursday

MEAL	PORTION SIZE	CARB CHOICES (number)
Breakfast		
Old-Fashioned Rolled Oats (page 70)	1 cup	1½
Breakfast Pinto Beans (page 52)	½ cup	1
Sweet cherries	1 cup	1
Walnuts	½ ounce (7 halves)	free
Milk/unsweetened soy or almond	½ cup	free
Ground Flaxseed (page 64)	1–2 tablespoons	free
Lunch		
Pasta e Fagioli (page 152)	1½ cups	3
Confetti Cornbread (page 181)	2-inch square	1
Garden salad	2 cups	free
Fat-Free Italian Dressing (page 108)	2 tablespoons	free
Apple Waldorf Salad (page 100)	½ cup	1
Dinner		
Southwest Soup (page 94)	1 cup	⅔
Tortilla Strips (page 205)	12 strips	free
Total Carb Choices		9⅙

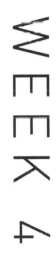

WEEK 4

Friday

MEAL	PORTION SIZE	CARB CHOICES (number)
Breakfast		
Fiesta Burrito (page 56)	1 burrito	1⅔
Pico Fresca (page 62)	½ cup	free
Breakfast Black Beans (page 50)	½ cup	1
Orange	1 medium	1
Almonds	½ ounce (11–12 nuts)	free
Ground Flaxseed (page 64)	1–2 tablespoons	free
Lunch		
Mazidra (page 147)	¾ cup	1
Mellow Brown Rice (page 194)	⅔ cup	2
Shredded lettuce	1½ cups	free
Diced tomatoes	¾ cup	free
Diced onions	3 tablespoons	free
Low-Fat Tofu Sour Cream (page 224)	2 tablespoons	free
Dill Cucumber Salad (page 107)	1 cup	½
Dinner		
White Bean and Kale Soup (page 97)	1 cup	1
Garden salad	2 cups	free
LCA Low-Sodium House Dressing (page 110)	2 tablespoons	free
Ezekiel 4:9 Sprouted Grain bread	1 slice	1
Smart Balance Light Buttery Spread	2 teaspoons	free
Total Carb Choices		9⅙

WEEK 4

Saturday

MEAL	PORTION SIZE	CARB CHOICES (number)
Breakfast		
Tofu Benedict (page 74)	1 serving	1⅓
Breakfast Great Northern Beans (page 51)	1 cup	2
Strawberries	1 cup	½
Pecans	½ ounce (10 halves)	free
Ground Flaxseed (page 64)	1–2 tablespoons	free
Lunch		
Savory Dinner Roast (page 157)	1 serving	⅔
Smashed Potatoes (page 201)	½ cup	1½
Windcrest Country Gravy (page 237)	¼ cup	free
Saucy Red Kidney Beans (page 188)	½ cup	1
Brussels sprouts	1 cup	free
Garden salad	2 cups	free
Creamy Ranch Dressing (page 104)	2 tablespoons	free
Holiday Pumpkin Pie (page 252)	1/16 pie	1
Dinner		
Cream of Celery Soup (page 85)	1 cup	1
Garden salad	2 cups	free
Fat-Free Italian Dressing (page 108)	2 tablespoons	free
Plum	1	½
	Total Carb Choices	9½

THINK ABOUT TAKING a trip in your car. In order to ensure that you get to your destination, you fill the gas tank at the beginning of your journey, not at the end. But most Americans have it backward when it comes to "fueling" their daily journeys. They typically skip breakfast and have their largest meal at the end of the day, when they're least likely to use that energy (sitting in front of the TV or computer, or reading before going to bed). That's a recipe for packing on the pounds through the dynamic of too-much-energy-in, not-enough-energy out.

At Lifestyle Center of America, we promote a simple lifestyle habit that can have a profound effect on your health. You remember your mom, a teacher, or a public service announcement advising you that "breakfast is the most important meal of the day"? Everybody seems to know this, but few people actually practice it. We feel it can be the key to the "miracle" touted in the title of our cookbook. So . . . *eat breakfast like a king, lunch like a prince, and supper like a pauper.*

In other words, you should eat more food earlier in the day and less food at the end of the day. If you really think about it, this "counterintuitive" idea starts to make sense. Food is energy—calories used as fuel to get you through the day. If you want the most energy to get you through the day, you should logically consume the most food earlier in the day—not at the end. Furthermore, eating big meals or snacks in the evening is a good way to make sure your morning blood sugar will be *high*, not low.

This prescription of eating most of your food early in the day holds true especially for people with weight to lose, and for people who want to conquer insulin resistance, the cause of type-2 diabetes. Eating a big breakfast is associated with successful weight loss maintenance in national studies, as well as by our own follow-up data. And people who eat the kind of breakfast foods we recommend—breakfast beans, old-fashioned rolled oats, and fresh, unsweetened berries—are sure to have better blood sugar responses than those eating traditional processed breakfasts, which are full of sugar, fat, and animal protein. Another added bonus: no hunger pangs a couple hours later like you get after a bowl of sugar-frosted cereal and a white bagel topped with jam. That's the reason there are no snack foods in this cookbook. You won't need them.

7-Grain Cereal Plus

Multigrain cereals are a dime a dozen, but this one's special because it contains soy grits, which makes it diabetic-friendly. And by the way, it tastes gr-r-r-reat.

3 cups water

½ teaspoon salt

1 cup Arrowhead Mills Seven Grain Hot Cereal

3 tablespoons whole flaxseed

■ Place all ingredients in a medium saucepan; bring to a boil. Reduce the heat, cover, and simmer, stirring occasionally until thick, 12 to 15 minutes.

▶ *Nutrition Note:* The whole flaxseed we add to this cereal provides fiber. To add healthy omega-3 fat, grind the seeds in a small coffee grinder (see Ground Flaxseed, page 64).

ANALYSIS FOR 1 SERVING:
½ cup

Calories: 91, Fat: 2.5 g, Total carbohydrates: 14.7 g, Protein: 4.0 g, Dietary fiber: 4.2 g, Sodium: 185 mg, Net carbs: 10.5 g, Carb Choice: ⅔

Alpine Muesli

A complete breakfast in a bowl, meusli is Switzerland's famous instant breakfast. We've adapted this recipe to be a diabetic-friendly quick breakfast in a bowl. Be sure to use unsweetened coconut.

¾ cup Toasted Oats (recipe below)

2 tablespoons chopped Toasted Walnuts (page 208)

1 medium apple, with peel, chopped

2 teaspoons dried cranberries

⅛ teaspoon ground cinnamon

1 teaspoon unsweetened shredded coconut

¾ cup unsweetened or plain soymilk

■ Place the oats and walnuts in a cereal bowl. Add the remaining ingredients. Stir together and serve.

ANALYSIS FOR 1 SERVING:
1⅔ cups

Calories: 469, Fat: 17.9 g, Total carbohydrates: 64.9 g, Protein: 17.6 g, Dietary fiber: 12.5 g, Sodium: 71 mg, Net carbs: 52.4 g, Carb Choice: 3½

Toasted Oats

MAKES 4 CUPS

4 cups old-fashioned rolled oats

■ Preheat the oven to 250°F. Spread the oats on an unsprayed baking sheet. Toast for 45 minutes, until golden brown. Cool before storing in a covered container.

Baked Apple Oats

A favorite of LCA guests, this fruity, chewy oatmeal bake takes the boredom of plain old oatmeal away.

¾ cup chopped apple with peel

1½ cups old fashioned rolled oats

2½ cups unsweetened or plain soymilk

½ teaspoon vanilla extract

½ teaspoon salt

½ teaspoon ground cinnamon

1 tablespoon unsweetened shredded coconut

¼ cup chopped walnuts

■ Preheat the oven to 350°F. Spread the apple on the bottom of an 8-inch-square baking dish. Distribute the oats evenly over the apples. Briefly whisk the soymilk, vanilla, salt, and cinnamon together, and pour slowly over the apples and oats. Sprinkle the coconut and walnuts on top. Bake for about 45 minutes, until golden brown.

ANALYSIS FOR 1 SERVING:
⅛ of recipe

Calories: 137, Fat: 5.1 g, Total carbohydrates: 18.1 g, Protein: 5.7 g,
Dietary fiber: 3.2 g, Sodium: 192 mg, Net carbs: 14.9 g, Carb Choice: 1

Breakfast Black Beans

Including beans is a top tip for a healthy, high-fiber, low-glycemic breakfast for people with diabetes. Make a big batch and store in the fridge for up to three days or in the freezer for up to a month for a quick breakfast side dish. Known also as "turtle beans," black beans have a matte black sheen, a creamy-colored flesh, and an earthy, rich flavor.

4 (15-ounce) cans regular-sodium black beans, drained (6 cups)

1½ cups water

1 teaspoon onion powder

½ teaspoon garlic powder

1 teaspoon ground cumin

1 teaspoon Red Star nutritional yeast flakes

■ Combine all the ingredients in a saucepan and heat through. Smash about ⅓ of the beans against the side of the pan to make thick and saucy beans. The beans can be refrigerated for up to 3 days or frozen for up to 1 month.

> **ANALYSIS FOR 1 SERVING:**
> ½ cup
>
> Calories: 136, Fat: 0.6 g, Total carbohydrates: 25.2 g, Protein: 8.4 g, Dietary fiber: 6.1 g, Sodium: 362 mg, Net carbs: 19.1 g, Carb Choice: 1

Breakfast Great Northern Beans

Great Northern beans are white beans that are larger than navy beans. They are so creamy when cooked that some people describe them as buttery. They run neck and neck with our Kickin' Western Chili (page 143) as the most popular breakfast bean dish served at Lifestyle Center of America.

4 (15-ounce) cans regular-sodium Great Northern beans, drained (6 cups)

1½ cups water

1 teaspoon onion powder

½ teaspoon garlic powder

1 teaspoon ground cumin

1 teaspoon Red Star nutritional yeast flakes

■ Combine all the ingredients in a saucepan and heat through. Smash about ⅓ of the beans against the side of the pan to make thick and saucy beans. The beans can be refrigerated for up to 3 days or frozen for up to 1 month.

ANALYSIS FOR 1 SERVING:
½ cup

Calories: 137, Fat: 0.4 g, Total carbohydrates: 24.7 g, Protein: 9.7 g, Dietary fiber: 6.2 g, Sodium: 235 mg, Net carbs: 18.5 g, Carb Choice: 1

Breakfast Pinto Beans

These very meaty-tasting beans are also called "Red Mexican" beans. They have streaks of reddish-brown on their skin, which disappear when they're cooked.

4 (15-ounce) cans regular-sodium pinto beans, drained (6 cups)

1½ cups water

1 teaspoon onion powder

½ teaspoon garlic powder

1 teaspoon ground cumin

1 teaspoon Red Star nutritional yeast flakes

■ Combine all the ingredients in a saucepan and heat through. Smash about ⅓ of the beans against the side of the pan to make thick and saucy beans. The beans can be refrigerated for up to 3 days or frozen for up to 1 month.

ANALYSIS FOR 1 SERVING:
½ cup

Calories: 131, Fat: 0.5 g, Total carbohydrates: 24.4 g, Protein: 7.9 g, Dietary fiber: 8.1 g, Sodium: 151 mg, Net carbs: 16.3 g, Carb Choice: 1

Cashew Burger Gravy

If you thought your gravy days were over because you're eating health-conscious, think again. Here's a mouthwatering, low-fat, very versatile gravy with high-fat flavor. Serve over Country Barley Biscuits (page 55) or Ezekiel 4:9 Sprouted Grain or other whole wheat toast.

1¾ cups water

¼ teaspoon salt

¼ cup raw cashew pieces

2 tablespoons cornstarch

1½ teaspoons McKay's Beef-Style Instant Broth and Seasoning, Vegan

6 tablespoons Morningstar Farms Grillers Recipe Crumbles, thawed then measured

1½ teaspoons dried chives

- Combine 1¼ cups of the water and the salt in a large saucepan and bring to a boil. In a blender, combine the cashews with the remaining ½ cup water, cornstarch, and beef-style seasoning, and blend until smooth and creamy, 1 to 2 minutes. Add the ingredients in the blender to the pan of boiling salted water, and cook, whisking, until gravy thickens. Add the crumbles and chives and cook, stirring, for 1 minute.

  ▶ *Nutrition Note:* This gravy is healthier than popular gravy because the fat from cashews is the healthier unsaturated kind, and the "burger" is not from ground beef. Besides ground beef's higher fat and saturated fat content, it's more likely to contain E. coli and other bacteria than other meat or plant-based ingredients.

ANALYSIS FOR 1 SERVING:
⅓ cup

Calories: 52, Fat: 3.0 g, Total carbohydrates: 5.0 g, Protein: 1.9 g,
Dietary fiber: 0.4 g, Sodium: 167 mg, Net carbs: 4.6 g, Carb Choice: ⅓

Chipped Tofu on a Shingle (CTOS)

Here's a plant-based twist on a famous military breakfast. Serve over Ezekiel 4:9 Sprouted Grain toast or a Country Barley Biscuit (opposite). Water-packed tofu comes in several different densities—soft, firm, or extra-firm. We use extra-firm in this recipe because it will keep its shape and not fall apart during the cooking process.

TOFU

1 cup water

3¾ teaspoons McKay's Chicken-Style Instant Broth and Seasoning, Vegan

2¼ teaspoons Red Star nutritional yeast flakes

¾ cup ¼-inch cubes water-packed, extra-firm tofu

SAUCE

1½ cups water

1½ tablespoons McKay's Chicken-Style Instant Broth and Seasoning, Vegan

¼ cup raw cashew pieces

¼ cup finely chopped onion

1 tablespoon low-sodium soy sauce

2 tablespoons cornstarch

- **For the tofu:** In a saucepan, combine the water, chicken-style seasoning, and nutritional yeast. Add the tofu to the saucepan and boil for 20 minutes. Set aside.
- **For the sauce:** In a blender, combine ¼ cup of the water, chicken-style seasoning, cashew pieces, onion, soy sauce, and cornstarch. Blend until smooth and creamy. Pour creamed mixture into a separate saucepan and add the remaining 1¼ cups of water. Bring to a boil, and cook, stirring constantly, until thick. Add the tofu mixture and stir gently.

ANALYSIS FOR 1 SERVING:
½ cup

Calories: 98, Fat: 5.3 g, Total carbohydrates: 8.1 g, Protein: 6.4 g,
Dietary fiber: 0.8 g, Sodium: 160 mg, Net carbs: 7.3 g, Carb Choice: ½

ANALYSIS FOR 1 SERVING:
½ cup on a shingle (1 slice Ezekiel 4:9 Sprouted Grain toast)

Calories: 178, Fat: 5.8 g, Total carbohydrates: 24.5 g, Protein: 9.6 g,
Dietary fiber: 2.6 g, Sodium: 234 mg, Net carbs: 21.9 g, Carb Choice: 1½

Country Barley Biscuits

The barley flour in these low-fat, diabetic-friendly gems gives them a unique, sweet, whole grain flavor. Make this generous batch and freeze some for future use.

¾ cup unsweetened soymilk, warmed to 110°F

1½ teaspoons rapid rise yeast

1 cup barley flour

1¼ cups whole wheat pastry flour

½ teaspoon salt

2 tablespoons plus 2 teaspoons canola oil

- Preheat the oven to the lowest temperature just to warm the oven, and turn the oven off. Briefly whisk together the soymilk and yeast and set aside. In a medium bowl, mix the dry ingredients together. Stir the oil into the yeast mixture, and stir into the dry ingredients. Stir quickly, but just enough that the ingredients come together. The dough should be moist, but hold together. The mixture will be sticky but fluffy. Turn out onto a well-floured board. Shape into a ball and roll out with a rolling pin to 1-inch thickness. Cut out biscuits using a 2-inch-round cutter.
- Spray a baking sheet with cooking spray. Place the biscuits, sides touching, on prepared baking sheet. Let rise in prewarmed oven for 30 minutes. Without removing from oven, turn the oven temperature to 350°F. Bake for 14 minutes, until golden brown.

ANALYSIS FOR 1 SERVING:
1 biscuit

Calories: 121, Fat: 3.7 g, Total carbohydrates: 19.5 g, Protein: 3.7 g,
Dietary fiber: 3.0 g, Sodium: 108 mg, Net carbs: 16.5 g, Carb Choice: 1

Fiesta Burrito

It will be a breakfast fiesta when your family or guests build their own healthy breakfast burrito using fixins you set out—try diced tomatoes, onions, peppers, and cilantro. In our Windcrest Restaurant we serve this burrito with guacamole or soy sour cream—but not both—to keep the fat down.

1 Ezekiel 4:9 Sprouted Grain tortilla

½ cup Traditional Scrambled Tofu (page 75) made with bell peppers and tomatoes

Salsa Fresca (page 229), Guacamole Rico (page 219), or Tofu Sour Cream Supreme (page 235)

Chopped raw vegetables of your choice

■ Heat the tortilla in a dry skillet on both sides until soft. Fill with scrambled tofu and roll up. Serve with salsa and vegetables.

ANALYSIS FOR 1 SERVING:
1 burrito with no toppings

Calories: 223, Fat: 7.5 g, Total carbohydrate: 30 g, Protein: 13.9 g, Dietary fiber: 4.3 g, Sodium: 398 mg, Net carbs: 25.7 g, Carb Choice: 1⅔

Flaxseed French Toast

MAKES 6 SLICES

This is a hearty, cholesterol-free version of the breakfast favorite typically laden with eggs and oil. The ground flaxseed provides heart-healthy omega-3 fat, and the Ezekiel 4:9 Sprouted Grain bread makes it diabetic-friendly, as long as you don't smother it with butter and maple syrup. Instead, top it with a dollop of Smart Balance Light Buttery Spread, sliced fruit, or our Very Berry Topping (page 77).

½ cup raw cashew pieces
1½ cups warm water
1½ tablespoons cornstarch
2 tablespoons whole flaxseed
1½ teaspoons vanilla extract

¼ teaspoon salt
⅛ teaspoon ground cinnamon or coriander
6 slices Ezekiel 4:9 Sprouted Grains bread or other whole-grain multigrain bread

■ In a blender on high setting, blend the cashews with ½ cup of the water until smooth and creamy, 1 to 2 minutes. Add the remaining ingredients, except for the bread, and blend on high speed until the mixture thickens. Pour into a shallow bowl or baking pan. Lightly spray a frying pan or griddle over medium heat with cooking spray. If using a griddle with a temperature gauge, set it at 350°F. Dip each slice of bread into the batter to coat the slice. Place in the frying pan and cook until golden brown on the bottom. Flip and brown the other side. Serve immediately.

▶ *Nutrition Note:* See Nutrition Note for Ground Flaxseed (page 64) to learn more about flaxseed.

> **ANALYSIS FOR 1 SERVING:**
> 1 slice with no toppings
>
> Calories: 126, Fat: 3.8 g, Total carbohydrates: 19.7 g, Protein: 4.5 g, Dietary fiber: 2.6 g, Sodium: 149 mg, Net carbs: 17.1 g, Carb Choice: 1

Golden Soy Oat Pancakes

MAKES 3 CUPS BATTER; 6 (2-PANCAKE) SERVINGS

They look and taste like traditional pancakes, but they won't raise your blood sugar like the original, thanks to the bean foundation. Add healthy toppings like fresh, low-glycemic fruit or Very Berry Topping (page 77).

Batter for Golden Soy Oat Waffles
(opposite)

■ Heat a skillet or griddle over medium heat and lightly spray with cooking spray. Drop ¼-cup portions of batter onto hot surface. Cook until browned on the bottom, flip, and brown the other side.

▶ *Nutrition Note:* See Nutrition Note for Golden Soy Oat Waffles (page 60).

ANALYSIS FOR 1 SERVING:
2 (4½-inch) pancakes

Calories: 160, Fat: 6.2 g, Total carbohydrates: 19.4 g, Protein: 8.0 g,
Dietary fiber: 3.8 g, Sodium: 198 mg, Net carbs: 15.6 g, Carb Choice: 1

Golden Soy Oat Waffles

MAKES 3 CUPS BATTER; 4 (6-INCH) WAFFLES

Waffles made of beans? Don't be surprised if you never go back to the flour-heavy originals. You won't taste the beans, but they give these waffles the right flavor and texture. And the best news is they make this breakfast very diabetic-friendly, because fiber-rich beans are one of the best plant foods for regulating blood sugar. If you don't want to use soybeans, you can substitute pinto, navy, Great Northern, cannellini, chickpea, or black beans in this recipe. Add healthy toppings like our Very Berry Topping (page 77), to taste. Sort dry beans, rinse in a colander, and place in a covered container in a generous amount of water, and refrigerate overnight (6 to 8 hours). In the morning, drain the beans and measure needed amount. One-half cup of any dry bean yields at least 1 cup after soaking. Store remaining soaked beans in fresh water in a covered container in the refrigerator for up to 10 days, changing the water once. You can soak a large batch of soybeans and freeze the extras in 1-cup portions for future waffle or pancake use. Thaw before using.

1 cup soaked soybeans

1⅔ cups water

1 tablespoon 100 percent natural floral honey

2 teaspoons canola oil

1 teaspoon vanilla extract or maple flavoring

½ teaspoon salt

1⅓ cups old-fashioned rolled oats

In a blender on the high setting, blend all the ingredients except the oats for a minimum of 90 seconds. Add the oats and blend for 1 minute. Pour the batter into a bowl and heat a regular (not Belgian) 6-inch-diameter waffle iron. By the time the waffle iron is fully heated, the batter will have thickened to the right consistency so no additional water will have to be added. Pour ¾ cup of the batter onto the waffle iron and close the lid. These whole grain–bean waffles are heavier and will require a longer cooking time, which varies with the brand of waffle iron and may take anywhere from 3 to 8 minutes. (You will need to experiment with your model of waffle iron.) Warning: Don't peek until the time is up, or the waffle will come apart.

▶ *Nutrition Note:* The combination of beans and grains in these waffles provides much more protein than average waffles. Most important, though, this recipe avoids the typically high-glycemic spike to your blood sugar caused by traditional waffles, and creates instead a nutritious, low-glycemic load, to help regulate your blood sugar at breakfast and keep you feeling satisfied for hours after eating (thanks to the fiber). Just don't smother these waffles with maple syrup!

ANALYSIS FOR 1 SERVING:
½ of a 6-inch waffle with no toppings

Calories: 109, Fat: 3.9 g, Total carbohydrates: 13.4 g, Protein: 5.7 g, Dietary fiber: 2.7 g, Sodium: 149 mg, Net carbs: 10.7 g, Carb Choice: ⅔

Santa Fe Waffles

*B*ring the taste of the Southwest to your breakfast table with this savory black bean waffle. Top with our Pico Fresca (page 62) for an authentic south of the border taste experience. In a pinch for time? Use low-sodium canned black beans, drained, instead of the soaked beans.

1 cup soaked black beans
1⅔ cups water
2 teaspoons canola oil
1 teaspoon onion powder
¼ teaspoon garlic powder

½ teaspoon salt
¼ teaspoon cayenne pepper
¼ teaspoon ground cumin
1⅓ cups old-fashioned rolled oats

■ In a blender on the high setting, blend all the ingredients except the oats for a minimum of 90 seconds. Add the oats and blend for 1 minute. Pour the batter into a bowl and heat a regular (not Belgian) 6-inch-diameter waffle iron. By the time the waffle iron is fully heated, the batter will have thickened to the right consistency so no additional water will have to be added. Pour ¾ cup of the batter onto the waffle iron and close the lid. These whole grain–bean waffles are heavier and will require a longer cooking time, which varies with the brand of waffle iron and may take anywhere from 3 to 8 minutes. You will need to experiment with your model of waffle iron. Warning: Don't peek until the time is up, or the waffle will come apart.

ANALYSIS FOR 1 SERVING:
½ of a 6-inch waffle

Calories: 94, Fat: 2.1 g, Total carbohydrates: 15.1 g, Protein: 4.1 g,
Dietary fiber: 2.9 g, Sodium: 149 mg, Net carbs: 12.2 g, Carb Choice: ⅔

Pico Fresca

This low-carb spicy topping combines vine-ripened tomatoes with avocado and a jalapeño chili. Add an extra jalapeño if you want more heat. Serve over Santa Fe Waffles (page 61). Remove jalapeño chili seeds with a knife, and be careful not to touch your eyes after touching the seeds. Wash your hands thoroughly.

1 cup ½-inch avocado chunks

1¼ cups coarsely chopped fresh tomato

3 tablespoons chopped onion

½ clove garlic, minced

1 tablespoon sliced jalapeño chili, seeds removed

2 tablespoons chopped fresh cilantro

¼ teaspoon salt

2 tablespoons fresh lime juice

■ Combine all the ingredients in a bowl.

ANALYSIS FOR 1 SERVING:
½ cup

Calories: 64, Fat: 4.8 g, Total carbohydrates: 5.8 g, Protein: 1.3 g,
Dietary fiber: 2.2 g, Sodium: 128 mg, Net carbs: 3.6 g, Carb Choice: free

---

Tac-Waffles

In this unusual recipe, we combine the kind of whole corn tortilla taste you'd associate with Mexican foods, into a traditional-looking waffle. The result is a lower-glycemic, full-flavor substitute for the original. Jazz it up with one of our delicious bean recipes and healthful toppings of your choice. Freeze extra waffles, and when in a pinch for time, pop the frozen waffles into the toaster for a quick and easy breakfast. Spread warm mashed beans on a toasted waffle. Then build as for a tostada, with diced tomato, onion, shredded lettuce, and avocado. Top with one of our delicious homemade salsas, like Salsa Fresca (page 229) or Chiapas Salsa (page 214).

⅓ cup raw sesame seeds

½ teaspoon salt

2 cups water

1¾ cups masa harina (available in Mexican section of the supermarket)

½ cup old-fashioned rolled oats

2 cups water

½ teaspoon vanilla extract

■ In a blender on high setting, blend the sesame seeds, salt, and water until creamy, 1 to 2 minutes. Add the remaining ingredients and blend for 1 minute. Pour the batter into a bowl and heat a regular (not Belgian) 6-inch-diameter waffle iron. Pour 1 cup of the batter onto the waffle iron, close the lid, and bake until lightly browned, 8 to 10 minutes, depending on the waffle iron. Warning: Don't peek until 8 minutes are up, or waffle will come apart.

ANALYSIS FOR 1 SERVING:
½ of a 6-inch waffle

Calories: 118, Fat: 3.8 g, Total carbohydrates: 18.4 g, Protein: 3.8 g, Dietary fiber: 2.9 g, Sodium: 122 mg, Net carbs: 15.5 g, Carb Choice: 1

Ground Flaxseed

MAKES: 3 TABLESPOONS PLUS 1½ TEASPOONS

Store your whole flaxseed in an airtight container in the refrigerator or freezer. We recommend you grind only as much as you need at one time for the optimal benefit. We encourage the daily use of ground flaxseed, a natural wonder for high-fiber, low-cholesterol health promotion.

2 tablespoons whole flaxseed, light or
  dark

■ Measure the seeds into a seed grinder, small coffee grinder, or mini food processor, and grind until fine, 10 to 30 seconds. Add to hot or cold cereal, breads, soups, or salads. Once ground, don't leave flaxseed at room temperature or it will spoil—always refrigerate or freeze in a sealed container, where it will keep for up to 6 months.

▶ *Nutrition Note:* Flaxseed is a good source of the essential omega-3 fatty acid called alpha-linolenic acid (ALA). ALA has many health benefits, including cell membrane health, indirect anti-inflammatory actions, and heart-protective abilities. ALA can be converted by the body into the long-chain-type of omega-3 fatty acid found in fish. This omega-3 fatty acid makes platelets less sticky and reduces inflammatory processes in blood vessels, thus decreasing the risk of a heart attack. The conversion of ALA to this long-chain omega-3 fatty acid is not very efficient, but every little bit helps.

Flaxseed is also a great source of dietary fiber, including a type of soluble fiber that helps lower cholesterol levels. It also provides protein, iron, and potassium. Flaxseed contains an impressive array of phytochemicals with powerful antioxidant and anti-cancer properties. One of these phytochemicals is a class of compounds called lignans, flaxseed being the leading dietary source. Lignans provide fiber; some are plant estrogens that protect against breast cancer.

Caution: As outstanding as flaxseed is, don't have more than 3 tablespoons whole seeds per day, because the husks of the seeds contain compounds that can be toxic in high doses.

ANALYSIS FOR 1 SERVING:
1 tablespoon ground flaxseed

Calories: 35, Fat: 2.4 g, Total carbohydrates: 2.4 g, Protein: 1.4 g,
Dietary fiber: 2 g, Sodium: 2 mg, Net carbs: 0.4 g, Carb Choice: free

---

Creamy Cranberry Quinoa

Quinoa (pronounced KEEN-wah) is a relative newcomer to the healthy American plate. It's usually associated with savory pilafs, but here it's used in a delicious new hot cereal option. Add healthy toppings to taste.

¾ cup quinoa

1½ cups water

¼ teaspoon salt

1 cup unsweetened or plain soymilk

¼ cup dried cranberries

1 teaspoon vanilla extract (optional)

■ Put the quinoa in a fine strainer and rinse under running water until the water runs clear. Drain well. In a medium saucepan, stir together the rinsed quinoa, water, and salt. Bring to a boil, reduce heat to low, cover, and simmer until the water is absorbed, 15 to 20 minutes. Stir in the soymilk, cranberries, and vanilla. Simmer until the cereal is thickened, 10 minutes.

► *Nutrition Note:* Quinoa, like buckwheat, is not a true grain, but it looks like one and can be used in similar ways, such as hot cereal, pilaf, and risotto. Though not apparent, quinoa's related to green leafy vegetables like spinach and Swiss chard. It's coated with a bitter-tasting resin (saponin), which protects the seeds from birds and insects, so before cooking always rinse quinoa in a fine strainer under running water until the water runs clear. Drain well and cook. For more on quinoa, see the Nutrition Note for Rustic Quinoa Pilaf (page 197). See Nutrition Note for Oatmeal Cranberry Cookies (page 257) and Wheat Berry Waldorf Salad (page 120) to learn about cranberries.

ANALYSIS FOR 1 SERVING:
½ cup with no sweetener or toppings

Calories: 120, Fat: 2.0 g, Total carbohydrates: 21.3 g, Protein: 4.3 g,
Dietary fiber: 2.1 g, Sodium: 128 mg, Net carbs: 19.2 g, Carb Choice: 1

Double Oats

We call this "double" oats because two different forms of oats are cooked together. The fine texture of oat bran complements the dense, chewy texture of steel-cut oats.

4 cups water
½ teaspoon salt

½ cup oat bran
1 cup steel-cut oats

■ Place all the ingredients in a medium saucepan and stir together. Bring to a boil, reduce the heat, cover, and simmer until thickened, stirring occasionally, 30 to 35 minutes.

▶ *Nutrition Note:* See Nutrition Notes for Old-Fashioned Rolled Oats (page 70) and Oat Bran Cereal (page 69) to learn about oats.

ANALYSIS FOR 1 SERVING:
½ cup

Calories: 106, Fat: 2.0 g, Total carbohydrates: 20.1 g, Protein: 4.9 g,
Dietary fiber: 3.5 g, Sodium: 170 mg, Net carbs: 16.1 g, Carb Choice: 1

Great Groats and Oats

"*Groats and oats*" *is shorthand for buckwheat groats and steel-cut oats. When we combined the buckwheat with steel-cut oats, the mild flavor of the oats was a perfect complement to the buckwheat, and it became a winner.*

½ cup buckwheat groats
½ cup steel-cut oats

¼ teaspoon salt
2½ cups water

■ Stir together all the ingredients in a medium saucepan and bring to a boil. Reduce heat, cover, and simmer, stirring occasionally, until the water is absorbed, 20 minutes.

▶ *Nutrition Note:* Buckwheat is not technically a grain—it's actually the fruit of a broadleaf plant belonging to the same family as sorrel and rhubarb. Buckwheat groats are the raw kernels of buckwheat. They contain protein (but not gluten), and are a notable source of iron, magnesium, and the B vitamin niacin.

ANALYSIS FOR 1 SERVING:
½ cup

Calories: 113, Fat: 1.4 g, Total carbohydrates: 22 g, Protein: 4.3 g,
Dietary fiber: 3.2 g, Sodium: 114 mg, Net carbs: 19 g, Carb Choice: 1

Hearty Barley Flakes

MAKES 4 CUPS; 8 (½-CUP) SERVINGS

This diabetic-friendly grain ranks as one of the most important cereal crops of the world because it grows well in a range of climactic conditions, from the highlands of Scotland to the deserts of Africa. Because of its health-promoting properties and low-glycemic index, we'd like to see it appear on more American breakfast tables.

4 cups water   ½ teaspoon salt
2 cups barley flakes

■ Stir all the ingredients together in a medium saucepan. Bring to a boil over medium heat, cover, reduce the heat, and simmer, stirring occasionally, until the water is absorbed, 15 to 20 minutes.

► *Nutrition Note:* Most people are familiar with the pearled form of barley. Unfortunately, pearl barley is refined, meaning it's been milled to remove the bran and most of the germ layers of the grain, resulting in the loss of the majority of its protein, vitamins, minerals, and some of its fiber. Barley flakes, on the other hand, like the rolled oats they resemble, are whole grain barley that's been flattened. As a whole grain, barley is a notable source of complex carbohydrates, thiamin, niacin, iron, the antioxidant mineral selenium, as well as fiber—particularly the soluble forms beta glucan and pectin, that help lower LDL (bad) cholesterol.

ANALYSIS FOR 1 SERVING:
½ cup cooked

Calories: 85, Fat: 0.3 g, Total carbohydrates: 18.7 g, Protein: 2.5 g,
Dietary fiber: 3.2 g, Sodium: 150 mg, Net carbs: 15.5 g, Carb Choice: 1

Oat Bran Cereal

A high-fiber reminder of smooth, old-fashioned farina when you top a piping-hot bowl with Smart Balance Light Buttery Spread, a pinch of cinnamon, and a teaspoon of low-glycemic sweetener.

3 cups water
¼ teaspoon salt

1 cup oat bran

■ Bring the water and salt to a boil in a medium saucepan over medium heat. Stir in the oat bran. Cover, reduce the heat, and simmer, stirring occasionally, for 3 to 5 minutes.

▶ *Nutrition Note:* Oats are famous for being rich in soluble fiber, especially a particular form of soluble fiber called beta glucan, found primarily in the oat bran. Beta glucan helps lower total cholesterol and LDL (bad) cholesterol levels. See Nutrition Note for Old-Fashioned Rolled Oats (page 70) to learn more about oats.

ANALYSIS FOR 1 SERVING.
1 cup with no toppings

Calories: 77, Fat: 2.2 g, Total carbohydrates: 20.8 g, Protein: 5.4 g,
Dietary fiber: 4.8 g, Sodium: 199 mg, Net carbs: 16 g, Carb Choice: 1

Old-Fashioned Rolled Oats

Good old-fashioned oatmeal is hard to beat—simple, inexpensive, very nutritious, easy to fix, and diabetic-friendly. Enjoy this all-time favorite at least twice a week. Overstirring during cooking causes oatmeal to become gummy.

4 cups water
¼ teaspoon salt

2 cups old-fashioned rolled oats

■ Bring the water and salt to a boil in a medium saucepan over medium heat. Stir in the oats. Reduce the heat, cover, and simmer, stirring occasionally, until the water is absorbed, 20 minutes.

▶ *Nutrition Note:* Who would have thought that ordinary oatmeal would be such a nutritional heavyweight? Oats are rich in complex carbohydrates and fiber, and have twice as much protein as brown rice. The fiber in oats is known to help regulate blood sugar and improve insulin sensitivity. Oatmeal contains good amounts of thiamin (a B vitamin), iron, selenium, magnesium, and zinc. Oats also contain phytochemicals, which help reduce the risk of heart disease. See the Nutrition Note for Oat Bran Cereal (page 69) to learn more about oats.

ANALYSIS FOR 1 SERVING:
1 cup

Calories: 156, Fat: 2.6 g, Total carbohydrates: 27.1 g, Protein: 6.5 g,
Dietary fiber: 4.3 g, Sodium: 150 mg, Net carbs: 22.8 g, Carb Choice: 1½

Simply Steel-Cut Oats

The dense, chewy texture of steel-cut oats is wonderful. Sprinkle with walnuts, and the desire for a crunchy, chewy hot breakfast cereal is more than adequately satisfied.

3 cups water

½ teaspoon salt

1 cup steel-cut oats

■ Bring the water and salt to a boil in a medium saucepan over medium heat. Stir in the oats. Reduce the heat, cover, and simmer, stirring occasionally, until the oats are tender and the water is absorbed, 40 to 45 minutes.

▶ *Nutrition Note:* Steel-cut oats are usually imported from Ireland or Scotland. They're made by cutting whole oat berries (called oat groats) into two or three pieces. They take longer to cook than rolled oats, but are definitely worth the wait. See Nutrition Notes for Old-Fashioned Rolled Oats (opposite) and Oat Bran Cereal (page 69) to learn more about oats.

ANALYSIS FOR 1 SERVING:
½ cup

Calories: 105, Fat: 1.7 g, Total carbohydrates: 18.3 g, Protein: 4.4 g,
Dietary fiber: 2.9 g, Sodium: 198 mg, Net carbs: 15.4 g, Carb Choice: 1

Walnut Wheat Berries

MAKES 3 CUPS; 6 (½-CUP) SERVINGS

Top with your favorite low-glycemic fruit. After cooking, the wheat berries will keep in the refrigerator for 3 to 4 days, or can be frozen for future use.

1 cup whole wheat berries

4 cups water

½ teaspoon salt

3 ounces walnuts (7 walnut halves per serving)

- **Slow Cooker Method:** The evening before you want to make this for breakfast, add the wheat berries, water, and salt to a slow cooker, and stir to combine. Cook on high for 2 hours. Turn to low and cook overnight. Top with walnuts.
- **Stovetop Method:** The evening before you want to make this for breakfast, add the wheat berries and 2 cups of the water to a bowl and soak in the refrigerator overnight. In the morning, combine the soaked berries, soaking water, the remaining 2 cups water, and the salt in a saucepan. Bring to a boil over medium heat, cover, reduce the heat, and simmer, stirring occasionally, until the water is gone and the wheat berries are tender, about 1½ hours. Top with walnuts.

▶ *Nutrition Note:* Wheat berries are rich in complex carbohydrates, fiber, thiamin, folate, Vitamin B_6, vitamin E, iron, selenium, magnesium, and zinc. They make a very diabetic-friendly hot cereal because their larger particle size slows down digestion, promoting a low-glycemic gradual release of glucose into the bloodstream. Walnuts are one of the richest sources of the essential omega-3 fatty acid, alpha-linolenic acid (ALA)—flaxseed and canola and soybean oils are others. Among other benefits, ALA helps prevent heart attacks. The monounsaturated and polyunsaturated fats in walnuts help lower blood cholesterol levels, especially when replacing saturated fat in the diet. Walnuts are also the top food source of melatonin, a powerful antioxidant that protects against heart disease and cancer, and helps regulate the sleep cycle. Good-quality protein, vitamin B_6, potassium, manganese, magnesium, zinc, and copper are just a few more nutritional benefits of walnuts.

ANALYSIS FOR 1 SERVING:
½ cup

Calories: 102, Fat: 0.6 g, Total carbohydrates: 21.8 g, Protein: 4.1 g,
Dietary fiber: 3.7 g, Sodium: 199 mg, Net carbs: 18.1 g, Carb Choice: 1

Whole Grain Corn Grits

Most corn grits are not whole grain—most of the bran is usually removed in the milling process. We like the added fiber, vitamins, and minerals found in whole grains, so we scoured the earth in search of a whole grain alternative. Thanks to Bob's Red Mill, we finally found one. Their whole grain (coarse-grind) cornmeal looks and tastes like traditional corn grits, and it's good for you, too. The grits may be topped with a teaspoon of Smart Balance Light Buttery Spread or our favorite, one serving of Pimiento Cheese Sauce (page 228).

2¼ cups water

¾ cup Bob's Red Mill whole grain cornmeal, coarse grind

¼ teaspoon salt

▪ Whisk together the water, cornmeal, and salt in a medium saucepan. Cover, bring to a boil over medium heat, reduce the heat to medium-low, and simmer, stirring occasionally, until thick, 15 to 20 minutes. Cover after each stirring.

> **ANALYSIS FOR 1 SERVING:**
> ½ cup with no toppings
>
> Calories: 72, Fat: 0.8 g, Total carbohydrates: 15.1 g, Protein: 1.9 g,
> Dietary fiber: 1.9 g, Sodium: 120 mg, Net carbs: 13.2 g, Carb Choice: 1

Tofu Benedict

*A*rnold was a traitor, but this recipe will not let you down. You won't miss the cholesterol and you won't miss the flavor or texture of original eggs Benedict. Chewy on the bottom, fluffy on the top, all smothered in gravy, this is a perennial favorite at LCA. Using leftover scrambled tofu and gravy makes this recipe quick and easy.

1 Ezekiel 4:9 Sprouted Grain English muffin or other 100 percent flourless English muffin

½ cup Traditional Scrambled Tofu (opposite)

⅔ cup Cashew Burger Gravy (page 53)

■ Slice the English muffin and toast. Assemble by placing ¼ cup of the scrambled tofu on each muffin half. Top each serving with ⅓ cup of the gravy. Serve immediately.

ANALYSIS FOR 1 SERVING:
1 Tofu Benedict

Calories: 173, Fat: 5.6 g, Total carbohydrates: 24.1 g, Protein: 8.9 g, Dietary fiber: 3.0 g, Sodium: 394 mg, Net carbs: 21.1 g, Carb Choice: 1⅓

Traditional Scrambled Tofu

Our non-egg take on traditional scrambled eggs is a big hit with our guests—especially those transitioning onto a plant-based diet. Season as you would eggs.

2 cups water-packed, extra-firm tofu

1½ teaspoons extra-virgin olive oil

½ cup chopped onion

¼ cup chopped bell pepper (optional)

½ cup fresh chopped tomatoes (optional)

2 tablespoons minced fresh green onion or dried chives

2 teaspoons McKay's Chicken-Style Instant Broth and Seasoning, Vegan

⅛ teaspoon turmeric powder

½ teaspoon salt

½ teaspoon onion powder

¼ teaspoon garlic powder

2 tablespoons Red Star nutritional yeast flakes

■ Remove the tofu from its package, rinse, drain, and set aside. Heat the olive oil in a large skillet over medium heat. Add the onion and other vegetables (if using) and sauté until tender, 3 to 4 minutes. Crumble the tofu into the vegetable mixture, stir in the remaining ingredients, and cook over medium heat for 5 to 10 minutes, stirring occasionally. Serve immediately.

▶ *Nutrition Note:* What is nutritional yeast? Yeast is a one-celled microorganism growth-form classified in the kingdom Fungi (the same family as edible mushrooms), which reproduces asexually by budding. Pure strains of *Saccharomyces cerevisiae* yeast are grown on mixtures of cane and beet molasses. After the fermentation process is completed, the yeast is harvested, thoroughly washed, pasteurized, and dried. We only use Red Star nutritional yeast, which is not made from by-products of breweries, distilleries, or paper mills, is not a genetically modified organism (GMO), and contains no added sugars or preservatives. Red Star nutritional yeast is grown specifically for its nutritional value. It provides protein, dietary fiber, B-complex vitamins—thiamin (B_1), riboflavin, (B_2), niacin (B_3), pyridoxine (B_6), cyanocobalamin (B_{12})—and folic acid. It's naturally low in fat and salt. Besides providing nutrition, Red Star nutritional yeast enhances the flavor and taste of whatever it's added to.

ANALYSIS FOR 1 SERVING:
½ cup without optional vegetables

Calories: 82, Fat: 4.4 g, Total carbohydrates: 5.0 g, Protein: 7.7 g,
Dietary fiber: 1.2 g, Sodium: 215 mg, Net carbs: 3.8 g, Carb Choice: free.

Western Omelet

Especially popular with kids, this home-on-the-range-flavored tofu dish is a great, low-carb way to start the day for any cowboy, pint-size or full-grown.

2 cups water-packed, extra-firm tofu, drained

6 tablespoons Pimiento Cheese Sauce (page 228)

1 teaspoon McKay's Chicken-Style Instant Broth and Seasoning, Vegan

⅛ teaspoon salt

¹⁄₁₆–⅛ teaspoon turmeric powder

¼ teaspoon garlic powder

2 tablespoons Red Star nutritional yeast flakes

¼ cup chopped green bell pepper

3 tablespoons chopped onion

½ cup chopped tomatoes

■ Preheat the oven to 350°F. Spray an 8-inch-square baking dish with cooking spray. Rinse the tofu, drain well, and mash into a bowl. Add the remaining ingredients and stir well. Transfer to prepared dish, cover, and bake for 20 minutes. Uncover and bake for 10 minutes.

ANALYSIS FOR 1 SERVING:
½ cup

Calories: 95, Fat: 4.9 g, Total carbohydrates: 6.0 g, Protein: 9.7 g,
Dietary fiber: 1.8 g, Sodium: 159 mg, Net carbs: 4.2 g, Carb Choice: ⅓

Very Berry Topping

The brilliant colors of berries make this sauce as beautiful as it is delicious. It's the perfect low-glycemic topping for waffles, pancakes, and desserts. For a nice flavor variation, add 1 tablespoon fresh lemon juice, ⅛ teaspoon orange extract, or ¼ teaspoon vanilla extract.

1 cup fresh sliced or frozen unsweetened strawberries, separated

½ cup fresh or frozen unsweetened blueberries

½ cup fresh or frozen unsweetened blackberries

½ cup fresh or frozen unsweetened sweet cherries

2 teaspoons 100 percent natural floral honey

■ Thaw berries if frozen. In a blender on high setting, blend ½ cup of the strawberries until creamy, about 1 minute. Pour into a bowl, add the remaining ingredients, and stir together. Serve over waffles as is or warm slightly in a saucepan or microwave before serving.

▶ *Nutrition Note:* Berries are part of the "miracle" of this cookbook. Nutritional wonders that make their sometimes high cost well worth every penny, berries are low-glycemic, and low in fat, calories, and sodium. They're also rich in fiber, potassium, vitamin C, and antioxidant phytochemicals that are potential cancer fighters and heart protectors.

ANALYSIS FOR 1 SERVING:
⅓ cup

Calories: 44, Fat: 0.4 g, Total carbohydrates: 10.8 g, Protein: 0.6 g, Dietary fiber: 2.3 g, Sodium: 2 mg, Net carbs: 8.5 g, Carb Choice: ½

SOUPS MAKE SENSE for people on a plant-based diet. Cold or hot, they're delicious, varied, and very filling when they're chock-full of beans, lentils, hearty vegetables, and heart-healthy whole grains. In this section, we offer a full gamut of our favorite soups, all of which—even our creamy soups—are totally free of unhealthy animal products, and all of which are low carb. The hallmark problem with soup in the Standard American Diet is a result of the high-sodium content of most canned soups, broth, and stocks. One-cup servings of our soups have about half the sodium—sometimes less—as typical commercial canned soups

These soups are all easy to prepare, and can all be made in bulk, frozen, or refrigerated, and reheated for multiple meals.

Remember our precept, "Breakfast like a king." We recommend eating the bulk of your calories early in the day, then skipping your evening meal, or at least eating light. For us, eating light means a small salad, a piece of fruit, and a cup of soup: That's all we serve our dinnertime guests at Windcrest Restaurant. And that's why we included our most hearty and filling stewlike soups in the entrées chapter instead of here.

Some of these recipes, like our Chickpea Noodle Soup and Cream of Asparagus Soup approximate familiar favorites, but without the meat and dairy. Others, like our Roasted Red Pepper Bisque and White Bean and Kale Soup might seem completely novel to you. We've also included some international soups, like Indian Lentil Soup and Gazpacho, to spice up your plant-based lifestyle, both literally and figuratively.

Feel free to experiment with plant-based, low-glycemic ingredients to create your own favorite soups: try quinoa, pearl barley, brown rice, squash, and a variety of above-the-ground vegetables, and remember to use vegetarian soup stock. Save the water from steamed vegetables and use it for your stock.

Butternut–Black Bean Soup

MAKES 2 QUARTS; 8 (1-CUP) SERVINGS

This is a Tex-Mex variation of a traditional butternut squash soup, made by adding high-fiber beans, cilantro, and onion.

5 cups 1-inch cubes peeled butternut squash

1 cup diced celery

½ cup diced onion

4 cups water

1 tablespoon McKay's Chicken-Style Instant Broth and Seasoning, Vegan

½ teaspoon salt

¹⁄₁₆ teaspoon cayenne pepper

1 (15-ounce) can low-sodium black beans, drained (1½ cups)

¼ cup chopped fresh cilantro

¼ cup chopped green onion

■ Add all ingredients except beans, cilantro, and onions to a pot, bring to a boil, and simmer, covered, until the squash is tender, about 1 hour. Remove from the heat. Blend with a stick (immersion) blender until creamy, or carefully transfer to a blender or food processor. Process on medium for 1 to 2 minutes. Return to the pot. Stir in the beans, cilantro, and green onion, and heat on low until hot.

▶ *Nutrition Note:* The deep orange color of butternut squash indicates the presence of the orange pigment beta carotene. The structure of beta carotene comprises two vitamin A molecules hooked together. Our bodies can split these apart, giving us two molecules of the essential nutrient vitamin A. Vitamin A has several very important functions in the body, the most famous of which, popularized by Bugs Bunny, is keen eyesight. As a phytochemical, beta carotene possesses antioxidant, immune-boosting, and cancer-fighting abilities. One cup of cooked butternut squash supplies 10 milligrams of beta-carotene. Butternut squash is also low in fat, high in fiber, and provides decent amounts of thiamin, niacin, Vitamin B_6, folate, vitamin C, magnesium, potassium, iron, and vitamin E. See Butternut Harvest Soup (page 82) to learn more about butternut squash.

ANALYSIS FOR 1 SERVING:
1 cup

Calories: 92, Fat: 0.4 g, Total carbohydrates: 20.1 g, Protein: 3.9 g,
Dietary fiber: 3.8 g, Sodium: 177 mg, Net carbs: 16.3 g, Carb Choice: 1

Butternut Harvest Soup

This golden soup suits a crisp autumnal day. Velvety and subtle, this quick and easy recipe gets a little extra zip from cayenne pepper. Butternut squash is one of the three most common winter squash found in American supermarkets, the other two being acorn and Hubbard. Winter squash are edible members of the gourd family. In contrast to summer squash, winter squash are harvested when they are mature and their skins are hard. This hard, protective skin gives winter squash a longer shelf life; some can be kept for months in a cool, dry place. See Nutrition Note for Butternut–Black Bean Soup (page 81) to learn more about butternut squash's nutritional benefits.

5 cups 1-inch cubes peeled butternut squash

1 cup diced celery

½ cup diced onion

4 cups water

1 tablespoon McKay's Chicken-Style Instant Broth and Seasoning, Vegan

½ teaspoon salt

1/16 teaspoon cayenne pepper

■ Place all the ingredients into a pot, bring to a boil, and simmer, covered, until the squash is tender, about 1 hour. Blend with a stick (immersion) blender until creamy, or carefully transfer to a blender or food processor and process on medium for 1 to 2 minutes. Return to the pot and reheat. Serve hot.

> **ANALYSIS FOR 1 SERVING:**
> 1 cup
>
> Calories: 48, Fat: 0.2 g, Total carbohydrates: 12.2 g, Protein: 1.1 g, Dietary fiber: 1.8 g, Sodium: 188 mg, Net carbs: 10.4 g, Carb Choice: ⅔

Chickpea Noodle Soup

This classic LCA soup is as comforting as the old-fashioned favorite, but without the unhealthy animal protein or high-carb processed noodles. Instead, garbanzos stand in for the chicken chunks, whole grain pasta provides the noodle, and chicken-style seasoning perfects the broth.

1½ teaspoons extra-virgin olive oil

½ cup chopped onion

1 clove garlic, minced

¼ cup minced carrot

3 tablespoons McKay's Chicken-Style Instant Broth and Seasoning, Vegan

3½ cups water

1 cup uncooked whole grain pasta

2 cups regular-sodium, canned chickpeas (garbanzos), drained

½ cup low-sodium canned diced tomatoes

1 tablespoon dried parsley

- Heat the olive oil in a large saucepan over medium heat. Add the onion, garlic, and carrot and sauté until the vegetables are tender, 4 to 5 minutes. Add the chicken-style seasoning, water, and pasta. Reduce the heat to medium-low, cover, and cook until the pasta is al dente, 10 to 15 minutes.
- Meanwhile, in a blender on medium, blend 1 cup of the chickpeas with the tomatoes until creamy, 1 to 2 minutes. Add the blended mixture and the remaining chickpeas and parsley to the saucepan, and heat until hot.

> **ANALYSIS FOR 1 SERVING:**
> 1 cup
>
> Calories: 149, Fat: 2.9 g, Total carbohydrates: 26 g, Protein: 6.4 g,
> Dietary fiber: 5.4 g, Sodium: 129 mg, Net carbs: 20.6 g, Carb Choice: 1⅓

Cream of Asparagus Soup

As soon as it gets wet and warm in spring, asparagus arrives. Its delicate flavor is featured in this lovely, pale green soup. No one will suspect its creaminess derives from blended potato and soymilk—they'll just ask for seconds of this low-calorie, low-fat, low-carb dish. If fresh asparagus is not available, use frozen.

2½ cups water

1 teaspoon McKay's Beef-Style Instant Broth and Seasoning, Vegan

1 teaspoon McKay's Chicken-Style Instant Broth and Seasoning, Vegan

1 cup diced, peeled red potato

1 cup sliced onion

½ cup chopped celery

4 cups ½-inch asparagus pieces

2 tablespoons cornstarch

2 cups unsweetened or plain soymilk

¼ teaspoon dried marjoram

1½ tablespoons Bragg Liquid Aminos

1 teaspoon salt

1/16 teaspoon cayenne pepper

■ In a large saucepan, bring the water and beef- and chicken-style seasonings to a boil. Add the potato, onion, and celery, and simmer for 15 minutes. Add the asparagus, and simmer for 15 minutes. Remove from the heat. Add the cornstarch and blend with a stick (immersion) blender until smooth, or cool and carefully transfer to a blender and process on medium for about 1 minute. Add the remaining ingredients, and simmer until the soup thickens. Serve hot.

▶ *Nutrition Note:* This elegant vegetable is a member of the lily family, and thus, is related to garlic, onions, and leeks. Asparagus contains an impressive array of phytochemicals, including beta-carotene, lutein, and rutin, which works with vitamin C to strengthen capillary walls. Asparagus is low in fat, high in fiber, and a respectable source of thiamin, riboflavin, niacin, vitamin B$_6$, vitamin C, potassium, and iron. Asparagus is also a super source of folate. Green asparagus is more flavorful and nutritious than white.

> **ANALYSIS FOR 1 SERVING:**
> 1 cup
>
> Calories: 83, Fat: 1.5 g, Total carbohydrates: 14.4 g, Protein: 4.5 g, Dietary fiber: 2.3 g, Sodium: 492 mg, Net carbs: 12.1 g, Carb Choice: 1

Cream of Celery Soup

This creamy soup is full-flavored with all the nuances of fresh celery and a whisper of cayenne pepper. This low-calorie, low-fat, low-carb soup makes a superlative starter for an elegant holiday menu, or a simple light supper meal when served with salad. Raw celery must be cut into ½-inch lengths before boiling to avoid stringiness in the finished soup.

2½ cups water

1 teaspoon McKay's Beef-Style Instant Broth and Seasoning, Vegan

1 teaspoon McKay's Chicken-Style Instant Broth and Seasoning, Vegan

1 cup diced, peeled red potato

1 cup sliced onion

½ cup chopped celery

4 cups ½-inch celery pieces

2 tablespoons cornstarch

2 cups unsweetened or plain soymilk

¼ teaspoon dried marjoram

1½ tablespoons Bragg Liquid Aminos

1 teaspoon salt

1/16 teaspoon cayenne pepper

■ In a large saucepan, bring the water and beef- and chicken-style seasonings to a boil. Add the potato, onion, and chopped celery, and simmer for 15 minutes. Add the celery pieces and simmer for 15 minutes. Remove from the heat. Add the cornstarch and blend with a stick (immersion) blender until smooth, or cool and carefully transfer to a blender. Blend on medium for about 1 minute. Add the remaining ingredients, and simmer until the soup thickens. Serve hot.

ANALYSIS FOR 1 SERVING:
1 cup

Calories: 79, Fat: 1.3 g, Total carbohydrates: 14.2 g, Protein: 3.5 g,
Dietary fiber: 2.6 g, Sodium: 542 mg, Net carbs: 11.6 g, Carb Choice: 1

Down-Home Green Pea Soup

Frozen peas make for easy prep in this high-fiber, high-vegetable-protein soup (and many expert chefs believe that flash-freezing gives them a stronger flavor than fresh peas, which lose oomph while traveling to the market). While this soup explodes with fresh pea taste, its vibrant green color is enhanced by "hidden" (blended) spinach.

1 teaspoon canola oil

2 cloves garlic, minced

2 medium onions, chopped

4½ cups water

1 tablespoon McKay's Chicken-Style Instant Broth and Seasoning, Vegan

4 cups frozen green peas

2 cups fresh spinach

¾ teaspoon salt

2 teaspoons Smart Balance Light Buttery Spread

1/16 teaspoon cayenne pepper (optional)

■ Heat the oil in a medium saucepan over medium heat. Add the garlic and onion and sauté until tender, 3 to 4 minutes. Add the water and chicken-style seasoning, and bring to a boil. Add the peas and cook for 1 to 2 minutes. Add the spinach and cook for 2 to 3 minutes. Stir in the salt, spread, and cayenne (if using). Blend the soup with a stick (immersion) blender until smooth, or cool and carefully transfer to a blender and puree on high for about 1 minute. Serve hot.

ANALYSIS FOR 1 SERVING:
1 cup

Calories: 86, Fat: 1.5 g, Total carbohydrates: 14.5 g, Protein: 4.4 g,
Dietary fiber: 4.8 g, Sodium: 345 mg, Net carbs: 9.7 g, Carb Choice: ⅔

Garden Minestrone Soup

The diverse flavors of a summer vegetable garden collaborate in our low-carb version of this satisfying Italian soup.

⅓ cup whole-grain elbow macaroni

1 teaspoon extra-virgin olive oil

⅓ cup diced onion

4 cups water

1 cup ½-inch carrot pieces

⅓ cup ½-inch celery pieces

1 cup ¼-inch zucchini pieces

1 cup diced canned tomatoes

1 cup low-sodium canned kidney beans, drained

1½ teaspoons McKay's Beef-Style Instant Broth and Seasoning, Vegan

1 teaspoon salt

1 teaspoon dried basil

½ teaspoon dried oregano

⅛ teaspoon garlic powder

1 bay leaf

- Cook the macaroni in plain boiling water (no oil or salt added), according to the package directions, until al dente and drain.
- Meanwhile, heat the oil in a saucepan over medium heat. Add the onion and sauté until tender, 3 to 4 minutes. Add the water, carrots, and celery and simmer until tender, about 15 minutes. Add the remaining ingredients, except the pasta, and simmer until the vegetables are tender, 15 to 20 minutes. Add the pasta and heat until hot. Remove the bay leaf and serve hot.

> **ANALYSIS FOR 1 SERVING:**
> 1 cup
>
> Calories: 89, Fat: 2.3 g, Total carbohydrates: 14.6 g, Protein: 3.9 g, Dietary fiber: 3.4 g, Sodium: 442 mg, Net carbs: 11.2 g, Carb Choice: ⅔

Gazpacho

Some days are just too hot for soup. This refreshingly chilled soup, popular across Spain in endless varieties, is like eating a cool tomato and pepper salad with a spoon—and it's just as low-carb and low-calorie. Gazpacho is traditionally served with various cold toppings: Try our Low-Fat Tofu Sour Cream (page 224) or Aioli (page 210) and some chopped avocado. You can use a food processor for all this chopping—just be sure not to puree all those veggies. Gazpacho requires the crunch of variegated, chopped vegetables.

1 small cucumber, peeled and finely chopped

1 clove garlic, minced

1 small yellow bell pepper, finely chopped

1 medium stalk celery, finely chopped

4 green onions, finely chopped

1 medium tomato, finely chopped

2 tablespoons chopped fresh cilantro

¼ cup finely chopped fresh parsley

½ teaspoon dried dill

¼ teaspoon ground dried thyme

1 teaspoon chopped fresh mint leaves

1 (14.5-ounce) can low-sodium diced tomatoes

2 tablespoons no-salt-added tomato sauce

1½ cups water

2 tablespoons McKay's Chicken-Style Instant Broth and Seasoning, Vegan

2 tablespoons fresh lime juice

2 teaspoons extra-virgin olive oil

½ teaspoon salt

10 tablespoons diced avocado

5 lime wedges

■ Place the vegetables, cilantro, parsley, dill, thyme, and mint in a large bowl and set aside. Process the canned tomatoes and tomato sauce in a food processor on medium setting for about 5 seconds, and add to the vegetables with the remaining ingredients. Mix together and chill well before serving. Serve cold, topped with 2 tablespoons diced avocado per serving and a lime wedge.

> **ANALYSIS FOR 1 SERVING:**
> 1 cup
>
> Calories: 91, Fat: 5.0 g, Total carbohydrates: 12.0 g, Protein: 2.1 g,
> Dietary fiber: 3.0 g, Sodium: 273 mg, Net carbs: 9 g, Carb Choice: ½

Indian Lentil Soup

The vivid red lentils in this soup cook down quickly to form a thick and savory puree, perfect for a cozy supper by the fire. Chili powder and parsley lend a taste of the subcontinent without overpowering the essential flavor of the lentils.

1 cup red lentils

5 cups water

1 clove garlic, crushed

1 tablespoon extra-virgin olive oil

1 cup chopped onion

½ cup thinly sliced celery

1 cup finely diced carrots

1 ½ tablespoons tomato paste

1 bay leaf

⅛ teaspoon chili powder

1 ½ teaspoons salt

1 ½ cups canned whole crushed tomatoes

½ cup chopped fresh parsley

■ Combine the lentils, water, garlic, olive oil, onion, celery, and carrots in a large saucepan, and bring to a boil. Cover, reduce the heat, and simmer, stirring occasionally, for about 1 hour. Add the remaining ingredients, except the parsley, and simmer for 10 minutes. Just before serving, stir in the parsley. Serve hot.

ANALYSIS FOR 1 SERVING:
1 cup

Calories: 120, Fat: 2.1 g, Total carbohydrates: 19.9 g, Protein: 7.1 g,
Dietary fiber: 6.9 g, Sodium: 550 mg, Net carbs: 13 g, Carb Choice: 1

Mediterranean Barley and Lentil Soup

We might have called this cinnamon-spiced specialty of the house "Ezekiel Soup," because its fiber-filled mainstays—lentils and barley—have been part of the Mediterranean diet since at least when Ezekiel (circa 600 BC) mentioned them in the Old Testament. If you can't find the mildly peppery French lentils this nourishing recipe calls for, use the more common brown ones.

6 cups water

½ cup French lentils

3 tablespoons pearl barley

2 teaspoons extra-virgin olive oil

¾ cup chopped onion

3 medium cloves garlic, minced

2 teaspoons ground cumin

½ teaspoon ground coriander

1⁄16 teaspoon cayenne pepper

¼ teaspoon salt

½ teaspoon onion salt

1 small cinnamon stick

1 cup plus 2 tablespoons low-sodium, canned diced tomatoes

1 tablespoon plus 2 teaspoons McKay's Chicken-Style Instant Broth and Seasoning, Vegan

- In a large soup pot, combine 1 cup of the water, the lentils, and barley. Bring to a boil, reduce the heat, and simmer, covered with the lid ajar, until the water is nearly gone, 20 minutes.
- While the lentils and barley are cooking, heat the olive oil in a medium skillet over medium heat. Add the onion and garlic and sauté until tender, 3 to 4 minutes. Add the onion and garlic to the soup pot, along with the remaining 5 cups water and the remaining ingredients. Bring to a boil, reduce the heat, and simmer for 40 minutes, covered with the lid ajar. Remove the cinnamon stick and serve hot.

ANALYSIS FOR 1 SERVING:
1 cup

Calories: 116, Fat: 2.1 g, Total carbohydrates: 20.1 g, Protein: 5.5 g,
Dietary fiber: 5.4 g, Sodium: 265 mg, Net carbs: 14.7 g, Carb Choice: 1

Our Favorite Split-Pea Soup

Abundant, buttery split peas create a satisfying, old-world flavor in this soup that's quick and easy, because split peas require no presoaking. This soup provides a high-fiber, high-vegetable-protein boost. To ensure the split peas are thoroughly cooked, be sure the pot is covered during the entire cooking time.

1 cup dry green split peas

4 cups water

½ cup ¼-inch celery pieces

½ cup ¼-inch carrot pieces

¼ cup ¼-inch onion pieces

1 tablespoon McKay's Chicken-Style Instant Broth and Seasoning, Vegan

2 tablespoons dried onion flakes

1 teaspoon extra-virgin olive oil

½ teaspoon salt

2 tablespoons Red Star nutritional yeast flakes

■ In a medium pot, bring the split peas and water to a boil. Cover, immediately reduce the heat, and simmer until the peas are half cooked, about 30 minutes. Add the remaining ingredients and simmer, covered, until tender, about 45 minutes. Serve hot.

ANALYSIS FOR 1 SERVING:
1 cup

Calories: 158, Fat: 1.4 g, Total carbohydrates: 27.5 g, Protein: 10.9 g, Dietary fiber: 9.9 g, Sodium: 274 mg, Net carbs: 17.6, Carb Choice: 1

Roasted Red Bell Pepper Bisque

In this sweet and robust soup, fire-roasted peppers are whizzed into a thick, brilliant red puree, one of Windcrest Restaurant's favorite soups. Top it with a dollop of tofu sour cream, and enjoy with a winter salad.

2½ cups water

1 teaspoon McKay's Beef-Style Instant Broth and Seasoning, Vegan

1 teaspoon McKay's Chicken-Style Instant Broth and Seasoning, Vegan

1 cup peeled, diced potatoes

1 cup diced onion

½ cup chopped celery

2½ cups jarred fire-roasted red bell peppers or canned pimientos, drained

2 tablespoons cornstarch

2 cups unsweetened or plain soymilk

¼ teaspoon dried marjoram

1½ tablespoons low-sodium soy sauce

1 teaspoon salt

1/16 teaspoon cayenne pepper

■ In a large saucepan, bring the water and beef- and chicken-style seasonings to a boil. Add the potatoes, onion, and celery, and simmer for 15 minutes. Add the bell peppers and simmer for 15 minutes. Remove from heat, add the cornstarch, and blend with a stick (immersion) blender until smooth, or cool and carefully transfer to a blender and blend on medium for about 1 minute. Add the remaining ingredients and simmer until the soup thickens. Serve hot.

ANALYSIS FOR 1 SERVING:
1 cup

Calories: 89, Fat: 1.4 g, Total carbohydrates: 16.6 g, Protein: 3.9 g, Dietary Fiber: 2.9 g, Sodium: 506 mg, Net carbs: 13.7 g, Carb Choice: 1

Sautéed Button Mushroom Soup

This is our full-flavor but "lighter" version of traditional cream of mushroom soup, made without dairy or butter. Even though it's significantly lower in sodium, it still tastes like the old, earthy favorite. For an even more intense flavor, try using wild mushrooms such as oyster, morel, or porcini—or a mix of your favorites.

⅓ cup raw cashew pieces

4½ cups water

3 tablespoons cornstarch

1 tablespoon McKay's Beef-Style Instant Broth and Seasoning, Vegan

¾ cup Morningstar Farms Grillers Recipe Crumbles, or other vegetarian burger crumbles, thawed

1 teaspoon salt

2 teaspoons Smart Balance Light Buttery Spread

1½ cups finely chopped onions

3 cups diced button or other mushrooms

1 tablespoon dried chives

■ In a blender on high, blend the cashews, 2 cups of the water, cornstarch, beef-style seasonings, and crumbles until smooth, 1 to 2 minutes. While the blender is running, combine the remaining 2½ cups of water and salt in a medium saucepan, and bring to a boil. Add blender mixture to the boiling water, and cook, stirring constantly with a whisk, 8 to 12 minutes, until thickened. Remove from heat and set aside.

■ Melt the spread in a small skillet over medium heat. Add the onions and sauté until tender, 3 to 4 minutes. Add the mushrooms to the onions, and cook until the mushrooms release and reabsorb their liquid. Add the mushrooms and chives to the cashew mixture in the saucepan, cover, and cook on low heat for 10 to 15 minutes. Serve hot.

ANALYSIS FOR 1 SERVING:
1 cup

Calories: 102, Fat: 4.7 g, Total carbohydrates: 12.0 g, Protein: 4.3 g, Dietary fiber: 1.7 g, Sodium: 525 mg, Net carbs: 10.3 g, Carb Choice: ⅔

Southwest Soup

Sweet corn and tangy tomatoes complement each other in this invigorating soup that's low-calorie, low-fat, and low-carb. At LCA, we serve this soup with a choice of healthful toppings: shredded red cabbage, chopped avocado, chopped tomato, chopped onion, diced radishes, black beans, and Tortilla Strips (page 205).

1 teaspoon extra-virgin olive oil
½ cup diced onion
¾ cup julienned carrot
⅓ cup thinly sliced celery
¼ cup diced yellow squash
1 teaspoon McKay's Beef-Style Instant Broth and Seasoning, Vegan

7 cups quartered fresh Roma tomatoes
1 cup water
½ cup frozen whole-kernel yellow corn
1 teaspoon salt
¼ cup chopped fresh cilantro

■ Heat the olive oil in a large saucepan over medium heat. Add the onion and sauté until tender, 3 to 4 minutes. Stir in the carrot, celery, squash, and beef-style seasoning. Process the tomatoes in a food processor until they are very soupy, with some small pieces. Add the tomatoes, water, corn, and salt to the soup. Simmer for 15 minutes. Stir in the cilantro just before serving.

ANALYSIS FOR 1 SERVING:
1 cup

Calories: 71, Fat: 1.5 g, Total carbohydrates: 14.7 g, Protein: 2.5 g,
Dietary fiber: 3.3 g, Sodium: 421 mg, Net carbs: 11.4 g, Carb Choice: ⅔

Spicy Vegetable Quinoa Soup

Quinoa is an ancient pseudo-grain of Aztec origin, which is now coming into its own in America's health-conscious culture. Sautéing the quinoa and whole cumin seeds intensifies the smoky cumin flavor, while the whole cloves add a startling punch. Rinse quinoa in a fine-mesh colander until the water becomes clear, to remove the bitter-tasting resin (saponin).

1 tablespoon extra-virgin olive oil

½ cup quinoa, rinsed and patted dry

2½ teaspoons cumin seed

1 teaspoon ground dried thyme

1¼ teaspoons dried oregano leaves

2 whole cloves

¼ cup chopped onion

1 cup chopped red bell pepper

2 cloves garlic, minced

1 jalapeño chili, seeds removed, minced

1 (14.5-ounce) can no-salt-added diced tomatoes

½ cup frozen whole-kernel yellow corn

1 teaspoon salt

7 cups low-sodium vegetable broth or 7 cups water and 5 tablespoons McKay's Chicken-Style Instant Broth and Seasoning, Vegan

1¾ cups regular-sodium canned cannellini beans or other white beans, drained

2 tablespoons chopped fresh cilantro leaves

■ Heat the olive oil in a large pot over medium heat. Add the quinoa and cumin seed, and cook for 2 to 3 minutes, stirring constantly. Add the thyme, oregano, whole cloves, onion, bell pepper, garlic, and jalapeño chili, and stir well. Add the canned tomatoes, corn, salt, broth, and beans, and bring to a boil. Reduce the heat and simmer uncovered until the quinoa is soft, about 20 minutes. Remove from the heat, stir in the cilantro, and serve hot.

ANALYSIS FOR 1 SERVING:
1 cup

Calories: 136, Fat: 2.6 g, Total carbohydrates: 24.1 g, Protein: 5.9 g,
Dietary fiber: 4.3 g, Sodium: 490 mg, Net carbs: 19.8 g, Carb Choice: 1⅓

Summer Vegetable Soup

A super-low-calorie, low-fat, and low-carb light and wholesome soup, this recipe is abundant with summer vegetables and a touch of thyme.

4 cups water

1⅓ cups cubed unpeeled red potatoes

1 cup sliced zucchini

1 cup sliced yellow squash

⅔ cup chopped fresh tomatoes

⅔ cup sliced celery

1⅓ cups sliced carrots

⅔ cup chopped onion

1 bay leaf

½ teaspoon garlic powder

1 teaspoon onion powder

1/16 teaspoon dried savory

½ teaspoon dried thyme

2 teaspoons McKay's Chicken-Style Instant Broth and Seasoning, Vegan

1 teaspoon salt

2 teaspoons Red Star nutritional yeast flakes

⅓ cup fresh spinach

⅓ cup frozen green beans

⅓ cup frozen green peas

2 tablespoons chopped fresh parsley

■ In a large pot, place all the ingredients, except the spinach, green beans, peas, and parsley, and bring to a boil. Reduce the heat, cover, and simmer until the vegetables are tender, about 20 minutes. Add the remaining ingredients, and return to a boil. Remove from the heat and serve immediately.

ANALYSIS FOR 1 SERVING:
1 cup

Calories: 55, Fat: 0.3 g, Total carbohydrates: 12.2 g, Protein: 2.2 g,
Dietary fiber: 2.9 g, Sodium: 330 mg, Net carbs: 9.3 g, Carb Choice: ½

White Bean and Kale Soup

We don't know whether anyone's ever done it before, but we've made this healthy medley of white beans and kale a local favorite.

1½ teaspoons extra-virgin olive oil

½ cup diced onion

1 clove garlic, minced

3 cups water

1 cup ¼-inch carrot pieces

6 tablespoons ¼-inch celery pieces

1 cup chopped fresh kale

⅛ teaspoon garlic powder

1½ teaspoons seasoned salt

⅛ teaspoon dried thyme

1 bay leaf

¼ teaspoon dried rosemary

1 cup regular-sodium canned diced tomatoes

1 tablespoon chopped fresh parsley

1 cup low-sodium canned white beans, drained

■ Heat the olive oil in a saucepan over medium heat. Add the onion and garlic and sauté under tender, 3 to 4 minutes. Add the water, carrot, celery, kale, and seasonings, and simmer, covered, until the vegetables are tender, about 15 minutes. Stir in the tomatoes, parsley, and beans, and simmer for 10 minutes. Remove the bay leaf before serving.

ANALYSIS FOR 1 SERVING:
1 cup

Calories: 96, Fat: 1.7 g, Total carbohydrates: 16.5 g, Protein: 4.9 g,
Dietary fiber: 4.3 g, Sodium: 504 mg, Net carbs: 12.2 g, Carb Choice: 1

I F YOU'RE ADOPTING a plant-based lifestyle, which we hope you are, you'll soon find you consider many of these salads more than mere accompaniments to a meal, but meals in themselves—at least sometimes. Don't be deceived by the delicate flavors of our seasonings and dressings, or the light touch of the vegetables and tofu that comprise our salads: Most of these dishes pack a mean nutritional punch, and their fiber content gives them bulk that will be filling, even if you don't follow with an entrée.

When it came to selecting salads for this cookbook, we followed the concept of "eating by color." That means you should eat a variety of vegetables daily, such as you would find in a salad, in order to ensure you're getting a good mix of vitamins, minerals, and phytochemicals.

We urge you to try our dressings, which are quick and easy to prepare, to ensure you're not pouring unnecessary sugar, salt, fat, calories, and preservatives onto otherwise healthy salads. We can recommend a few commercial brands, such as our favorite, Wish-Bone Olive Oil Vinaigrette. Other good choices are Wish-Bone Balsamic Vinaigrette, Newman's Own Light Raspberry and Walnut Dressing, Kraft Light Done Right! Raspberry Vinaigrette, or Annie's Naturals Low Fat Gingerly Vinaigrette. You can use other dressings as long as they meet the following criteria: no animal products, no wine, 5 or less grams of fat per serving, 5 or less grams of sugar per serving, 300 milligrams or less sodium per serving, and no NutraSweet or Splenda. Remember to watch your dressing portions.

Apple Waldorf Salad

This is our low-fat, nondairy version of the famed Waldorf salad originally created at the Waldorf-Astoria Hotel in New York City.

¼ cup Toasted Walnuts (page 208)

3 cups diced apples, such as Gala, Fuji, Pink Lady, Golden Delicious, or other sweet variety

½ cup raisins

1 cup diced celery

¾ cup Low-Fat Tofu Mayonnaise (page 223)

1½ teaspoons fresh lemon juice

1½ tablespoons 100 percent natural floral honey

⅛ teaspoon salt

■ Place the walnuts, apples, raisins, and celery in a bowl. In a separate bowl, mix together the mayonnaise, lemon juice, honey, and salt and stir into the salad. Cover and refrigerate until chilled.

ANALYSIS FOR 1 SERVING:
½ cup

Calories: 114, Fat: 4.1 g, Total carbohydrates: 19.6 g, Protein: 2.2 g, Dietary fiber: 2.2 g, Sodium: 121 mg, Net carbs: 17.4 g, Carb Choice: 1

Caesar Salad

We toss crisp Romaine lettuce with our robust Caesar Salad Dressing in this healthy version of the popular salad. If making ahead, keep dressing and lettuce separated and well-chilled. Toss together with croutons right before serving. This salad is best when served on a chilled plate.

6 cups coarsely chopped romaine lettuce
½ cup thinly sliced red onion
¼ cup pitted black olives

1 cup Crunchy Croutons (page 106)
½ cup Caesar Salad Dressing (page 102)

■ Place the lettuce, onion, olives, and croutons in a bowl. Add the dressing and toss well.

ANALYSIS FOR 1 SERVING:
1 cup

Calories: 61, Fat: 3.3 g, Total carbohydrates: 6.0 g, Protein: 3.2 g,
Dietary fiber: 1.8 g, Sodium: 180 mg, Net carbs: 4.2 g, Carb Choice: free

---

Caesar Salad Dressing

*O*ur *dressing tastes a lot like the original, but without the eggs, anchovies, and excess oil that pack on the pounds and cholesterol. You can find citric acid in the canning section of the supermarket.*

½ cup Low-Fat Tofu Mayonnaise (page 223)

2 tablespoons canola oil

2 tablespoons fresh lemon juice

2 cloves garlic, minced

2 tablespoons Red Star nutritional yeast flakes

½ teaspoon salt

¼ teaspoon citric acid

■ Combine all the ingredients in a bowl and stir together well. Cover and refrigerate until serving, storing separately from salad ingredients until time to serve. The dressing will keep in the refrigerator for up to 3 days.

ANALYSIS FOR 1 SERVING:
2 tablespoons

Calories: 52, Fat: 4.4 g, Total carbohydrates: 1.9 g, Protein: 2.2 g,
Dietary fiber: 0.6 g, Sodium: 195 mg, Net carbs: 1.3 g, Carb Choice: free

---

Cauliflower-Broccoli Salad

This distinctly American combo—sweet, chunky, chewy, and spirited—is a breeze to prepare, and ideal for a summer barbecue or lunchtime side dish. Save time by chopping the cauliflower and broccoli in a food processor. The pieces should be slightly larger than a grain of rice.

2 cups finely chopped cauliflower

1 cup finely chopped broccoli florets

½ cup diced red apple

2 tablespoons raw sunflower seeds

2 tablespoons dried cranberries

¼ cup Nayonaise spread

1½ teaspoons fresh lemon juice

¹⁄₁₆ teaspoon salt

2 tablespoons frozen apple juice
    concentrate, thawed

1 pinch cayenne pepper

■ Mix all ingredients together in a medium bowl. Cover and refrigerate until ready to serve.

▸ *Nutrition Note:* Cauliflower and broccoli, members of the cruciferous vegetable family, are laden with potential cancer-fighting phytochemicals. Broccoli is a true nutritional superstar: It abounds in fiber, folate, vitamin C, riboflavin, potassium, and iron. It's also a fair source of protein and calcium.

Broccoli also contains the carotenoids beta-carotene and lutein. Besides providing vitamin A for the body, beta carotene has antioxidant and anticancer properties. Lutein is found in the macula of the human retina, so lutein in broccoli is believed to protect against age-related macular degeneration. Cauliflower, too, packs a nutritional punch. It's an outstanding source of vitamin C, and a good source of folate and vitamin B_6. To preserve as much vitamin C as possible, be sure to steam cauliflower lightly or eat it uncooked, as in this salad.

ANALYSIS FOR 1 SERVING:
½ cup

Calories: 58, Fat: 3.0 g, Total carbohydrates: 7.4 g, Protein: 1.5 g,
Dietary fiber: 1.6 g, Sodium: 87 mg, Net carbs: 5.8 g, Carb Choice: ⅓

Creamy Ranch Dressing

Ranch dressing remains popular, even among those who've adopted a plant-based diet. No problem if you substitute soy mayonnaise and soymilk for the dairy ingredients. You get a low-fat, lower-sodium, full-flavor ranch dressing that's just as creamy and so much better for you.

1½ cups Low-Fat Tofu Mayonnaise (page 223)

½ cup unsweetened or plain soymilk

2 tablespoons Creamy Ranch Dry Mix (opposite)

■ Stir all the ingredients together well in a small bowl. Cover and refrigerate until serving. The dressing will keep in the refrigerator for up to 3 days.

ANALYSIS FOR 1 SERVING:
2 tablespoons

Calories: 25, Fat: 1.6 g, Total carbohydrates: 1.5 g, Protein: 1.4 g,
Dietary fiber: 0.2 g, Sodium: 171 mg, Net carbs: 1.3 g, Carb Choice: free

---

Creamy Ranch Dry Mix

MAKES 2½ CUPS

*J*ust *two tablespoons of this mix with some Low-Fat Tofu Mayonaise (page 223) and soymilk will make a healthy nondairy version of ranch dressing, one of the most popular dressings at LCA. Once the dry mix is made, you can make fresh batches of ranch dressing for months.*

15 Kavli thin crispbread
½ cup dried minced onion
2 tablespoons dried dill weed
2 cups dried parsley

¼ cup onion salt
¼ cup garlic salt
¼ cup onion powder
¼ cup garlic powder

■ Pulse the crispbread, minced onion, and dill in a food processor until powdery, 2 to 3 minutes. Add the parsley and pulse a few times, making sure not to turn the parsley into powder. Pour into a small bowl, add the remaining ingredients, and stir together. The mix will keep in a covered container for up to 6 months.

Crunchy Croutons

Croutons with a garlic, onion, and herb bite might seem like a thing of the past if you're trying to control your blood sugar. But if you use low-glycemic, whole-grain bread like Ezekiel 4:9, and watch your portions, you can tumble these babies on your Caesar Salad (page 101) or other salads, and rest assured they're diabetic-friendly. The croutons store well in an airtight container.

12 slices Ezekiel 4:9 Sprouted Grain or other whole grain bread with crusts, cut into ½-inch cubes

1 tablespoon extra-virgin olive oil

1½ tablespoons onion powder

1½ tablespoons garlic powder

1½ teaspoons dried oregano leaves

2 teaspoons dried basil

1 tablespoon dried parsley

½ teaspoon salt

■ Preheat the oven to 225°F. Place the bread in a bowl. Add the remaining ingredients and gently toss together well. Spread on a baking sheet and bake, turning every 10 minutes, for a total of 40 minutes, until completely dry.

ANALYSIS FOR 1 SERVING:
½ cup

Calories: 81, Fat: 2.1 g, Total carbohydrates: 11.5 g, Protein: 4.8 g, Dietary fiber: 1.8 g, Sodium: 157 mg, Net carbs: 9.7 g, Carb Choice: ⅔

Dill Cucumber Salad

If you love the distinctive zing of dill, this cool salad will revitalize you on a hot and lazy summer day—with practically no calories.

1¾ cups ½-inch cucumber cubes

1 cup ½-inch tomato pieces

¼ cup ¼-inch red onion pieces

⅛ teaspoon celery seed

½ teaspoon dried dill weed

⅛ teaspoon salt

⅛ teaspoon garlic powder

½ cup Tofu Sour Cream Supreme (page 235) or Tofutti Better Than Sour Cream

■ Place the vegetables in a medium bowl. Stir the seasonings and the Tofu Sour Cream Supreme together, add to the vegetables, and mix well. Cover and refrigerate until ready to serve.

▶ *Nutrition Note:* Cucumbers belong to the same vegetable family as pumpkin, zucchini, watermelon, and other squash. Because of their high water content (96 percent of their weight is water), cucumbers are among the lowest-calorie vegetables. Because of all that water, cucumber's nutritional content is also low, though they do contain high potassium levels. The surprisingly interesting nutritional fact about cucumbers is that their skin is a good source of lutein, a cartenoid phytochemical found in the macula of the human retina: Consuming them can combat macular degeneration.

ANALYSIS FOR 1 SERVING:
½ cup made with Tofu Sour Cream Supreme

Calories: 46, Fat: 2.6 g, Total carbohydrates: 5.2 g, Protein: 1.2 g,
Dietary fiber: 0.9 g, Sodium: 118 mg, Net carbs: 4.3 g, Carb Choice: free

ANALYSIS FOR 1 SERVING:
½ cup made with Tofutti Better Than Sour Cream

Calories: 34, Fat: 1.6 g, Total carbohydrates: 5.1 g, Protein: 0.8 g,
Dietary fiber: 0.9 g, Sodium: 91 mg, Net carbs: 4.2 g, Carb Choice: free

---

Fat-Free Italian Dressing

We make our quick and easy Italian dressing fat free without adding a lot of carbs, as commercial brands do, by substituting fructose-sweetened lemon juice for vinegar.

1 (0.7-ounce) package Good Seasons Italian dressing mix

2 tablespoons plus 2 teaspoons fresh lemon juice

1 cup water

1 teaspoon fructose

1½ teaspoons Resource ThickenUp food thickener or other instant thickener

▧ Blend all the ingredients together in a blender on high for about 20 seconds. Let stand for 10 minutes and serve or refrigerate.

ANALYSIS FOR 1 SERVING:
2 tablespoons

Calories: 8, Fat: 0.01 g, Total carbohydrates: 2.1 g, Protein: 0.02 g,
Dietary fiber: 0.02 g, Sodium: 269 mg, Net carbs: 2.1 g, Carb Choice: free

---

Green Soybean Salad

This recipe spotlights the flavorful and super-nutritious edamame bean. Water chestnuts add crunch to this salad, and the red bell pepper a punch of color. Serve as a starter, side, or entrée.

1½ cups shelled fresh or frozen green soybeans (edamame)
½ cup frozen whole-kernel yellow corn
¼ cup ¼-inch red bell pepper pieces
¼ cup ¼-inch red onion pieces
¼ cup finely chopped fresh parsley
½ cup canned sliced water chestnuts

½ teaspoon salt
2½ tablespoons fresh lemon juice
2 teaspoons fructose
½ teaspoon garlic powder
½ teaspoon dried basil
½ teaspoon extra-virgin olive oil

■ Steam the soybeans in a steamer basket set over 1 inch of water for 5 minutes. Add the corn and steam for 5 minutes. Rinse the soybeans and corn in a colander under cold running water. Drain and place in a medium bowl. Add the remaining ingredients and mix well. Cover and chill before serving.

▶ *Nutrition Note:* Also known as edamame, green soybeans were developed to be picked and used in their immature stage so they could be consumed fresh. That means the cooking time is much less than for mature, dried beans. Edamame have a mild flavor and are rich in complex carbohydrates, fiber, protein, and the good, unsaturated kind of fat. The protein in soybeans is high quality, equal to that of beef, minus the saturated fat, cholesterol, and calories. Edamame also contain notable amounts of thiamin, riboflavin, vitamin C, folate, calcium, iron, and magnesium.

ANALYSIS FOR 1 SERVING:
½ cup

Calories: 128, Fat: 4.5 g, Total carbohydrates: 16.2 g, Protein: 8.4 g,
Dietary fiber: 3.8 g, Sodium: 278 mg, Net carbs: 12.4 g, Carb Choice: 1

LCA Low-Sodium House Dressing

The idea behind a good dressing is to complement salad—not overwhelm it. The popular house dressing at our Windcrest Restaurant has a mild and beguiling flavor, not unlike traditional Thousand Island dressing, though, of course, without the dairy. You can use this as a dip, too—just omit the water.

½ cup mild picante sauce

¼ cup water

¼ teaspoon salt

2 tablespoons canola oil

½ (12.3-ounce) carton Mori-Nu lite, firm silken tofu

1½ tablespoons fresh lemon juice

½ teaspoon 100 percent natural floral honey

■ Blend ¼ cup of the picante sauce with the remaining ingredients in a blender on high setting until creamy, about 1 minute. Pour into a bowl and stir in the remaining ¼ cup picante sauce. Cover and refrigerate until chilled before serving.

ANALYSIS FOR 1 SERVING:
2 tablespoons

Calories: 23, Fat: 1.8 g, Total carbohydrates: 0.98 g, Protein: 0.8 g,
Dietary fiber: 0.2 g, Sodium: 84 mg, Net carbs: 0.7 g, Carb Choice: free

---

No-Oil Raspberry Dressing

Lemon juice provides the acidity that makes this dressing taste like authentic vinaigrette. It's fat-free and low-calorie, but watch your portion size because the fruit juice that gives this dressing its raspberry zing can affect your blood sugar (it's concentrated, after all).

3 (0.7-ounce) packages Good Seasons Italian dressing mix

½ cup plus 1 tablespoon fresh lemon juice

2 cups water

6 tablespoons raspberry–white grape juice frozen concentrate

⅓ cup Resource ThickenUp or other instant food thickener

■ Blend all ingredients in a blender on high until smooth, about 20 seconds. Chill in covered container until ready to serve. Dressing will keep in the refrigerator for up to 10 days.

ANALYSIS FOR 1 SERVING:
2 tablespoons

Calories: 21, Fat: 0.0 g, Total carbohydrates: 5.2 g, Protein: 0.1 g,
Dietary fiber: 0.1 g, Sodium: 314 mg, Net carbs: 5.1 g, Carb Choice: ⅓

Pea and Peanut Salad

A classic from LCA's kitchens, our Pea and Peanut Salad is all about the crunch. A favorite with kids, this one's perfect for picnics and sunny-day parties for grown-ups, too, when a crisp and energizing salad hits the spot. Experiment with spices: We like adding 2 teaspoons dried mint leaves or 1 teaspoon curry powder.

1½ cups frozen green peas

½ cup canned julienne-style water chestnuts, drained

¼ cup chopped onion

2 tablespoons lightly roasted salted peanuts

1 tablespoon lightly roasted sunflower seeds, unsalted

1 tablespoon pumpkin seeds

¼ teaspoon garlic and herb seasoning (salt-free)

¼ teaspoon onion salt

⅛ teaspoon garlic salt

2 tablespoons chopped red bell pepper

1 tablespoon plus 1 teaspoon Tofutti Better Than Sour Cream or LCA Basic Tofu Sour Cream (page 220)

Rinse and drain frozen peas and place in a bowl. Add the remaining ingredients and mix together well. Chill in a covered container before serving.

ANALYSIS FOR 1 SERVING:
½ cup with Tofutti Better Than Sour Cream

Calories: 90, Fat: 4 g, Total carbohydrates: 10.1 g, Protein: 3.9 g, Dietary fiber: 2.9 g, Sodium: 177 mg, Net carbs: 7.2 g, Carb Choice: ½

ANALYSIS FOR 1 SERVING:
½ cup with LCA Basic Tofu Sour Cream

Calories: 8.1, Fat: 4.1 g, Total carbohydrates: 8.3 g, Protein: 4.0 g, Dietary fiber: 2.7 g, Sodium: 162 mg, Net carbs: 5.4 g, Carb Choice: ⅓

South-of-the-Border Black Bean Salad

MAKES 4¾ CUPS; ABOUT 9 (½-CUP) SERVINGS

Every plant-based gourmet knows the ideal fresh salad covers all the sensory bases: It's packed with vibrant and diverse tastes, textures, and colors. That's why this low-calorie black bean salad is one of our finest. Dappled with the archetypal Southwestern hues of black, gold, green, and red, this salad satisfies with multifaceted flavors and textures, too, from soft avocado to chewy and vigorous pimiento, from the bite of onion to the yield of ripe tomato.

1 (15-ounce) can regular-sodium black beans, drained (1½ cups)

1 cup frozen whole-kernel yellow corn

½ cup chopped green onion

½ cup minced green bell pepper

½ cup peeled, pitted, diced avocado

1 (2-ounce) jar diced pimientos, drained (¼ cup)

½ cup chopped fresh tomatoes

¼ cup chopped fresh cilantro

¼ cup Fat-Free Italian Dressing (page 108)

1 tablespoon fresh lime juice

½ cup sliced black olives, drained

⅛ teaspoon garlic powder

- In a large bowl, toss all the ingredients together. Cover, refrigerate until chilled, and serve.

ANALYSIS FOR 1 SERVING:
½ cup

Calories: 52, Fat: 2.3 g, Total carbohydrates: 13.6 g, Protein: 3.4 g, Dietary fiber: 3.3 g, Sodium: 320 mg, Net carbs: 10.3 g, Carb Choice: ⅔

Strawberry-Spinach Salad

The enthralling juxtaposition of garlic, spinach, and strawberries, all bathed in a healthy raspberry dressing, makes this summer salad vanish from the salad bowl so much faster than a run-of-the-mill salad. For a low-fat, lower-sodium commercial dressing, use Newman's Own Light Raspberry and Walnut Dressing.

15 cloves garlic, peeled

¼ cup Toasted Pecans (page 207)

⅓ cup No-Oil Raspberry Dressing (page 111)

12½ cups packed baby leaf spinach

½ cup thinly sliced red onion

1½ cups sliced strawberries or sliced fresh pears (with peel)

■ Preheat the oven to 300°F. Roast the garlic by placing cloves in a foil pouch and spraying for 3 seconds with cooking spray. Seal the pouch and bake for 10 to 12 minutes. Toss all the ingredients together in a large bowl and serve immediately.

> **ANALYSIS FOR 1 SERVING:**
> 1½ cups
>
> Calories: 76, Fat: 3.8 g, Total carbohydrates: 9.9 g, Protein: 2.8 g,
> Dietary fiber: 3.2 g, Sodium: 181 mg, Net carbs: 6.7 g, Carb Choice: ½

Sunburst Salad

This sparkly citrus salad is much beloved by our guests, many of whom have told us they make a meal out of it. It's classy and bold, and just the thing for impressing guests or pampering yourself and your family in a healthy way. Keep dressing and lettuce separate and well-chilled. Toss together just before serving. Serve on a chilled plate.

3 tablespoons Low-Fat Tofu Mayonnaise (page 223)

1½ tablespoons Tofu Sour Cream Supreme (page 235)

2 tablespoons frozen orange juice concentrate, thawed

1 teaspoon grated orange zest

1 (8-ounce) bag Morningstar Farms Meal Starters Veggie Chik'n Strips

1 large kiwifruit, peeled, thinly sliced

⅓ cup canned mandarin orange segments, drained

⅓ cup finely chopped celery

1 tablespoon 100 percent natural floral honey

¼ teaspoon salt

8 cups torn medium pieces romaine lettuce

2 tablespoons Toasted Cashews (page 206)

■ In a medium bowl, stir together the Low-Fat Tofu Mayonnaise, Tofu Sour Cream Supreme, orange juice concentrate, and orange zest. Add the Chik'n Strips, kiwifruit, oranges, celery, honey, and salt. Toss to coat. Cover and refrigerate for 2 hours. Before serving, add the lettuce and cashews, and toss gently until completely mixed.

ANALYSIS FOR 1 SERVING:
1½ cups

Calories: 119, Fat: 3.9 g, Total carbohydrates: 13.1 g, Protein: 10 g, Dietary fiber: 2.3 g, Sodium: 392 mg, Net carbs: 10.8 g, Carb Choice: ⅔

Tabouli Salad

*T*his classic grain salad juxtaposes the intoxicating flavors of lemon, green onions, and mint to recollect the mystery and tumult of the Middle East.

½ cup bulgur wheat

1 cup hot water

¼ cup chopped fresh parsley, without stems

⅔ cup ¼-inch green onion pieces

1½ cups ¼-inch peeled cucumber pieces

1½ cups ¼-inch tomato pieces

1 clove garlic, minced

½ teaspoon salt

3 tablespoons fresh lemon juice

2 tablespoons extra-virgin olive oil

¾ teaspoon dried mint (optional)

▪ Bring the bulgur and water to a boil in a saucepan. Cover the pan and gently boil until the water is absorbed, 15 minutes. The bulgur will be fluffy. Transfer to a bowl, cover, and refrigerate until chilled. Add the remaining ingredients to the bulgur, toss to combine, and serve.

▶ *Nutrition Note:* You may be wondering what the differences are between wheat bulgur and cracked wheat. Cracked wheat is, as its name implies, whole wheat berries or kernels that have been "cracked" or ground into coarse, medium, or fine pieces for faster cooking (about 15 minutes as opposed to over an hour to cook whole wheat kernels). Wheat bulgur is a processed form of cracked wheat. The whole wheat berries are first steam-cooked and then dried. Then the whole kernels are "cracked" or ground into coarse, medium, or fine pieces. Wheat bulgur requires less cooking time than cracked wheat because it has been precooked during the steaming process. In fact, you can just soak it in hot water to rehydrate it.

ANALYSIS FOR 1 SERVING:
¾ cup

Calories: 100, Fat: 4.9 g, Total carbohydrates: 13.5 g, Protein: 2.4 g,
Dietary fiber: 3.3 g, Sodium: 209 mg, Net carbs: 10.2 g, Carb Choice: ⅔

Tofu Cottage Cheese

MAKES 2 CUPS; 8 (¼-CUP) SERVINGS

*T*his recipe is a vegetarian chameleon. Thanks to the curdlike crumbles of stark-white tofu and the tang of citric acid, it looks, smells, and tastes much like regular cottage cheese, but without the baggage and ill effects of dairy—and with very little carb. You can use it however you use regular cottage cheese—mixed with fruit or stuffed in a whole wheat pita, for example. Or you can use it in recipes as you would use ricotta cheese, such as lasagne, our Gourmet Eggplant Stacks (page 136), or our Party Pasta Bake (page 149). Transform the flavor of your Tofu Cottage Cheese with the flick of a wrist by changing the seasonings. Dried basil and garlic offer an Italian flair, but you can use chili powder, curry, turmeric, dill, or anything else you can imagine.

2 cups water-packed, extra-firm tofu, drained and crumbled

½ teaspoon salt

1⅛ teaspoons onion powder

⅛ teaspoon garlic salt

1/16 teaspoon citric acid powder (see page 276)

1 tablespoon dried chives, basil, parsley, or a mix (optional)

6 tablespoons Tofu Sour Cream Supreme (page 235), LCA Basic Tofu Sour Cream (page 220), or Tofutti Better Than Sour Cream

■ Place the tofu in a bowl. Add the remaining ingredients and mix well. Cover and refrigerate until chilled before serving.

> **ANALYSIS FOR 1 SERVING:**
> ¼ cup with Tofu Sour Cream Supreme
>
> Calories: 65, Fat: 4.3 g, Total carbohydrates: 3.0 g, Protein: 4.9 g, Dietary fiber: 0.4 g, Sodium: 214 mg, Net carbs: 2.6 g, Carb Choice: free
>
> **ANALYSIS FOR 1 SERVING:**
> ¼ cup with LCA Basic Tofu Sour Cream
>
> Calories: 57, Fat: 4.0 g, Total carbohydrates: 1.4 g, Protein: 5.0 g, Dietary fiber: 0.2 g. Sodium: 202 mg, Net carbs: 1.2 g, Carb Choice: free
>
> **ANALYSIS FOR 1 SERVING:**
> ¼ cup with Tofutti Better Than Sour Cream
>
> Calories: 72, Fat: 4.5 g, Total carbohydrates: 4.6 g, Protein: 4.8 g, Dietary fiber: 0.6 g, Sodium: 227 mg, Net carbs: 4.0 g, Carb Choice: free

Tofu Greek Salad

This snappy salad is a perfect accompaniment to a veggie burger like Aunt Vienna's Mushroom and Black Bean Burger (page 131), our 10-Minute Burger (page 125), or a whole wheat pita pocket stuffed with Chunky Chickpea Spread (page 215). Cucumbers, onions, and black olives lend this salad its Greek character, and tofu cubes stand in as low-fat, low-calorie alternatives to traditional feta cheese.

1 cup water-packed, extra-firm tofu, drained

1 cup fresh tomato, cut into wedges

2 cups 1-inch-thick peeled cucumber slices

¼ cup diced red onion

½ cup pitted whole black olives

½ cup Fat-Free Italian Dressing (page 108) or other fat-free, low-sodium dressing

Leaf lettuce

■ Cut the tofu into ½-inch cubes and place in a bowl. Add the tomato, cucumber, onion, and olives. Add the dressing and toss to combine. Cover and refrigerate until chilled before serving. Serve on a bed of leaf lettuce.

> **ANALYSIS FOR 1 SERVING:**
> ¾ cup
>
> Calories: 62, Fat: 3.5 g, Total carbohydrates: 5.3 g, Protein: 4.2 g,
> Dietary fiber: 1.2 g, Sodium: 264 mg, Net carbs: 4.1 g, Carb Choice: free

Tomato, Cucumber, and Avocado Salad

You can make this simple but lively little side salad in a jiffy.

1½ cups 1-inch fresh tomato chunks

1½ cups 1-inch peeled cucumber chunks

¼ cup chopped onion

½ cup sliced black olives

½ cup 1-inch avocado chunks

¼ cup Fat-Free Italian Dressing (page 108)

Combine all the ingredients in a bowl and toss to coat with the dressing. Cover and refrigerate until serving.

> *Nutrition Note:* Here's an intriguing fact about avocados: Besides monounsaturated fat, avocados contain a phytochemical called beta-sitosterol, which helps lower cholesterol levels. Beta-sitosterol is a plant sterol, the plant equivalent of cholesterol in animals. Plant sterols are very similar to cholesterol in structure, so they compete with cholesterol for absorption from the digestive tract into the body. The end result is that beta-sitosterol keeps some cholesterol from being absorbed—and that means lower cholesterol levels in the bloodstream. Beta-sitosterol also has cancer-fighting properties. See Nutrition Note for Guacamole Rico (page 219) to learn more about avocados.

ANALYSIS FOR 1 SERVING:
½ cup

Calories: 39, Fat: 2.5 g, Total carbohydrates: 4.4 g, Protein: 0.8 g,
Dietary fiber: 1.4 g, Sodium: 145 mg, Net carbs: 3.0 g, Carb Choice: free

---

Wheat Berry Waldorf Salad

*C*risp, sweet-tart apples are married to the chewy goodness of wheat berries, mingled with cranberries and walnuts in this one-of-a-kind LCA salad.

6 tablespoons Low-Fat Tofu Mayonnaise (page 223) or Nayonaise spread

2 cups cooked wheat berries (see page 9)

1¼ cups chopped apple (with peel)

1 cup chopped celery

6 tablespoons chopped walnuts

6 tablespoons dried cranberries

2 tablespoons fresh lemon juice

¼ teaspoon salt

2 tablespoons fructose

■ Combine all the ingredients in a large bowl, and mix together well. Cover and refrigerate until ready to serve.

► *Nutrition Note:* Native to North America, cranberries were used by Native Americans for medicinal purposes and as a dye for rugs, blankets, and clothes. More than 100 cultivated varieties of cranberries have largely replaced the wild ones. Most cranberries are grown in Wisconsin and Massachusetts, though New Jersey is "bogged-down" as well. Only 10 percent of the commercial crop is sold fresh, and the rest is used in juice or canned cranberry sauce. While cranberries are low in fat, calories, and protein, they are a good source of fiber and vitamin C. Cranberries are especially rich in several potent, health-promoting phytochemicals. The red anthocyanin, from which they derive their color, has heart-protective antioxidant properties: It appears to reduce the oxidation of LDL ("bad") cholesterol, and reduce platelet clumping, which reduces one's risk of developing heart attack–inducing blood clots. Benzoic acid is another phytochemical with strong antioxidant effects, while ellagic acid and epigallo-catechin gallate (EGCG) are cancer-fighting compounds. See Nutrition Note for Oatmeal-Cranberry Cookies (page 257) to learn more about cranberries. See Nutrition Note for Walnut Wheat Berries (page 72) to learn about wheat berries.

ANALYSIS FOR 1 SERVING:
½ cup made with Low-Fat Tofu Mayonnaise

Calories: 135, Fat: 5.1 g, Total carbohydrates: 20.7 g, Protein: 2.9 g, Dietary fiber: 2.1 g, Sodium: 132 mg, Net carbs: 18.6 g, Carb Choice: 1

ANALYSIS FOR 1 SERVING:
½ cup made with Nayonaise

Calories: 138, Fat: 7.1 g, Total carbohydrates: 17.3 g, Protein: 2.4 g, Dietary fiber: 1.7 g, Sodium: 173 mg, Net carbs: 15.6 g, Carb Choice: 1

Zippy Kale Salad

*K*ale is rarely used raw because of its too-intense flavor, but our soy-lemon marinade tones down its bitterness (the longer it sits, the better), and helps make this salad a hit at potlucks and picnics. The secret to this salad is to cut the kale finely, chiffonade style, making sure that you have no large pieces. Also, mix often so that the marinade is distributed evenly over the vegetables.

2½ tablespoons fresh lemon juice

2 tablespoons Bragg Liquid Aminos

½ teaspoon onion powder

¼ teaspoon garlic powder

2½ tablespoons water

1½ teaspoons extra-virgin olive oil

3 cups finely chopped fresh kale, stems removed

¾ cup thinly sliced radishes

1 Roma tomato, diced

¼ cup diced red bell pepper

2 medium green onions, chopped

2½ tablespoons raw sunflower seeds

■ In a small bowl, whisk together the lemon juice, Bragg Liquid Aminos, onion powder, garlic powder, water, and olive oil. Place the kale in a medium bowl. Add the dressing and remaining ingredients and mix well. Cover and refrigerate for at least 1 hour before serving.

▶ *Nutrition Note:* Kale is a member of the cruciferous vegetable family, which includes broccoli, Brussels sprouts, cauliflower, collard greens, mustard greens, rutabagas, turnips, and watercress. These vegetables are named cruciferous, derived from the Latin word for "cross," because they bear cross-shaped flowers. Kale provides fiber, vitamin K, vitamin C, vitamin B_6, and iron. Two cups of cooked kale also contains close to 200 milligrams of calcium—two-thirds the amount in a cup of cow's milk with only 72 calories and 1 gram of fat! Many greens contain substances called oxalates, which prevent calcium from being absorbed; the classic example is spinach. Fortunately, kale has low oxalate levels, making its calcium more available. Kale is also richly endowed with several antioxidant, cancer-fighting phytochemicals. See Nutrition Note for Brilliant Kale with Red Pepper and Onion (page 177) to learn more about this exceptional green.

ANALYSIS FOR 1 SERVING:
1 cup

Calories: 67, Fat: 4.3 g, Total carbohydrates: 5.8 g, Protein: 3.3 g,
Dietary fiber: 2.1 g, Sodium: 276 mg, Net carbs: 3.7 g, Carb Choice: free

---

ENTRÉES

I T'S PATENTLY UNTRUE that people on a plant-based diet eat mere "rabbit food" like celery sticks and dandelions for their main meals. The "miracle" of foods with high-complex carbs, high-fiber, and no unhealthy animal proteins or fats, means you can eat hearty but healthy meals that will keep your belly full, without filling you with guilt or harmful ingredients.

A few caveats, though: An important pillar of The 30-Day Diabetes Miracle is that these entrées are meant to be eaten earlier in the day than you might be used to. Ideally, you won't wait until after work to enjoy them but instead have them for your lunchtime meal, then eat much less, or nothing, for dinner. Part of our goal of ensuring most of these recipes are quick and easy is accomplished if you prepare the more "gourmet" entrées in advance, freeze them in appropriate portion sizes, then divvy them up for the family to take to work or school. Keep this new, healthier habit going on the weekends, too, by serving larger meals earlier in the day.

Second, we want to say a quick word about portion sizes. Even healthful foods become less healthful if you overindulge. As you transition onto a plant-based diet, stick to the portion sizes we recommend in the recipes. If you're eating at work or school, apportion the right size into transportable containers. If you're eating at home, serve from the kitchen, not the table. Check your temptation to overeat by eating more slowly, savoring your food. Eat a salad with lots of greens and above-the-ground vegetables with every entrée. The "miracle" works in three main ways:

- Usually, the high fiber content of ingredients in these meals will keep you much more satisfied than meals on the Standard American Diet.
- The whole grains and low-processing of ingredients means you won't get those hunger-inducing sharp spikes and drops in your blood sugar.
- No meat or dairy generally means less concentration of calories and fat.

That's a recipe for eating less volume of food yet feeling even more full, keeping your blood sugar under control, and losing weight. All that and it tastes great, too.

10-Minute Burger

Want a healthy burger right away? This veggie burger can be made in 10 minutes, start to finish.

1 Boca Vegan Meatless Burger or Morningstar Farms Vegan Burger

1 Ezekiel 4:9 Sprouted Grain burger bun

Low-Fat Tofu Mayonnaise (page 223) and/or mustard of your choice

1 to 2 dark green lettuce leaves

1 tomato slice

1 to 2 slices red onion

2 slices fresh avocado (⅛ of an avocado or ⅛ cup) (optional)

Preheat an ungreased, nonstick skillet over medium heat. Place frozen burger in a skillet and cook for 4 minutes on each side. Assemble with burger fixings and enjoy.

Nutrition Note: This burger will be about 2½ carb choices because it's one carb choice for each half of the bun. To decrease the carbs, make it an open-face burger. But from a health perspective, it would be better to have this veggie burger with the whole bun than a regular hamburger, even without the bun. Why? Because ground beef, most of which ends up in burgers, is one of the most harmful foods in the Standard American Diet. It's the second biggest source of saturated fat for the average American adult (after cheese, which people usually put on their burger, too). Ground beef can, misleadingly, be labeled "80 percent lean" or even "90 percent lean." Those claims are not allowed on other foods unless they are low in fat. Beef that is 90 percent lean is still 10 percent fat by weight, and that fat contributes 50 percent of the total calories!*

ANALYSIS FOR 1 BOCA VEGAN MEATLESS BURGER:
1 patty

Calories 39, Fat: 0.5 g, Total carbohydrates: 6 g, Protein: 13 g, Dietary fiber: 4 g, Sodium: 280 mg, Net carbs: 2 g, Carb Choice: free

ANALYSIS FOR 1 MORNING STAR FARMS VEGAN BURGER:
1 patty

Calories: 100, Fat: 2.5 g, Total carbohydrates: 7 g, Protein: 12 g, Dietary fiber: 4 g, Sodium: 280 mg, Net carbs: 3 g, Carb Choice: free

---

*Source: UC Berkeley Wellness Letter, June 2007.

Alfredo Sauce and Sautéed Mushrooms over Zucchini Ribbons

MAKES 1 SERVING

Our friend Brenda, a plant-based gourmet cook, shared the foundation of this recipe with us. Removing the dairy and substituting thinly sliced ribbons of zucchini for the pasta makes this rich-tasting entrée surprisingly healthful and diabetic-friendly.

1 cup Zucchini Ribbons (recipe below)   ¼ cup Sautéed Mushrooms (opposite)
¼ cup Alfredo Sauce (page 211)

■ Arrange the zucchini on a plate, top with the sauce and mushrooms, and serve hot or cold.

> **ANALYSIS FOR 1 SERVING:**
> 1 cup zucchini ribbons, ¼ cup Alfredo Sauce, and ¼ cup Sautéed Mushrooms
>
> Calories: 136, Fat: 6.9 g, Total carbohydrates: 14.3 g, Protein: 7.6 g,
> Dietary fiber: 3.9 g, Sodium: 410 mg, Net carbs: 10.4 g, Carb Choice: ⅔

Zucchini Ribbons

MAKES 7 CUPS

4 (8-inch-long) zucchinis

■ Peel the skin from the zucchini and discard. Continue peeling down to the seeds. Keep turning the zucchini as you peel to create thin, delicate ribbons, about ½-inch wide. (One 8-inch-long zucchini yields about 1¾ cups ribbons.)

> **ANALYSIS FOR 1 SERVING:**
> 1 cup
>
> Calories: 16, Fat: 0.2 g, Total carbohydrates: 3.3 g, Protein: 1.3 g,
> Dietary fiber: 1.4 g, Sodium: 3 mg, Net carbs: 1.9 g, Carb Choice: free

Sautéed Mushrooms

MAKES 2 CUPS; 8 (¼-CUP) SERVINGS

2 tablespoons Smart Balance Light Buttery Spread

5 cups sliced mushrooms

2 tablespoons low-sodium soy sauce

2 tablespoons fresh lime juice

1 clove garlic, minced

■ Melt the spread in a small skillet over medium heat. Add the mushrooms and sauté until tender, 3 to 4 minutes. Add the remaining ingredients and cook for 1 minute.

ANALYSIS FOR 1 SERVING:
¼ cup

Calories: 25, Fat: 1.4 g, Total carbohydrates: 2.3 g, Protein: 1.5 g, Dietary fiber: 0.6 g, Sodium: 156 mg, Net carbs: 1.7 g, Carb Choice: free

---

Armenian Lentil-Stuffed Peppers

MAKES 6 SERVINGS, ½ STUFFED PEPPER EACH

*O*ur peppers are stuffed with Armenian pilaf, which marries lentils with bulgur wheat and a hint of thyme.

3 large bell peppers (green, red, yellow, or a mixture)

1 tablespoon extra-virgin olive oil

1 cup thinly sliced onion

¼ cup dry lentils

1½ cups water

6 tablespoons bulgur or cracked wheat

¾ teaspoon salt

1 teaspoon onion powder

¼ teaspoon garlic powder

6 tablespoons Pimiento Cheese Sauce (page 228)

■ Preheat the oven to 350°F. Cut peppers in half lengthwise and scoop out seeds and ribs. Put cut side down in a baking dish filled with ¼-inch cold water. Place on a rack in a large pan and steam over boiling water for about 6 minutes. Remove the peppers with tongs and place on a paper towel to drain.

■ Heat the olive oil in a large saucepan over medium heat. Add the onion and sauté until tender, 3 to 4 minutes. Add the remaining ingredients, except the sauce, and cook until all the liquid is absorbed and the lentils are tender, about 35 minutes. Stuff each pepper with ⅓ cup of the lentil mixture. Top each pepper half with 1 tablespoon of the sauce. Bake for 30 minutes, until the peppers are soft.

▶ *Nutrition Note:* See Tabouli Salad (page 116) to learn what wheat bulgur and cracked wheat are, and how they differ.

ANALYSIS FOR 1 SERVING:
1 stuffed pepper half

Calories: 120, Fat: 3.6 g, Total carbohydrates: 19.0 g, Protein: 5.0 g,
Dietary fiber: 4.4 g, Sodium: 382 mg, Net carbs: 14.6 g, Carb Choice: 1

Baked Falafels

In our version of this classic Middle Eastern favorite, traditional spices are combined with chickpeas, and topped with a bold garlic sauce that makes it irresistibly good and surprisingly healthful for people with diabetes—especially because it's baked and not fried.

2 (15-ounce) cans regular-sodium chickpeas, drained (3 cups)

1½ cups water-packed, extra-firm tofu, drained

2 cloves garlic, minced

6 tablespoons finely chopped onion

1½ tablespoons chopped fresh parsley

1½ tablespoons chopped fresh cilantro

¼ cup low-sodium soy sauce or Bragg Liquid Aminos

1½ teaspoons ground cumin

⅜ teaspoon ground coriander

¾ slice Ezekiel 4:9 Sprouted Grain bread

4 Ezekiel 4:9 Prophet's pocket bread or other whole grain pita bread

8 tablespoons Garlic Tahini Sauce (page 218)

Chopped lettuce, tomatoes, cucumbers, or other vegetable toppings

■ Preheat the oven to 350°F. Lightly spray a baking sheet with cooking spray. Puree the chickpeas in a food processor or mash by hand in a large bowl. Rinse the tofu in a colander, mash, and add to the chickpeas. Add the garlic, onion, parsley, cilantro, soy sauce, cumin, and coriander, and mix together well. Break the bread slice into a dry blender, and process into crumbs. Pour into a small bowl.

■ To make the falafels, form balls using 2 tablespoons of the chickpea mixture. Roll the balls in bread crumbs, and place on prepared baking sheet. Bake for 25 to 30 minutes, until golden brown and firm. Put 2 falafel balls in half of a pocket bread, and top with 1 tablespoon sauce and toppings of choice.

▶ *Nutrition Note:* These Middle Eastern favorites are a wonderful source of protein in one of its most delicious forms. Unfortunately, falafels are traditionally prepared by frying or deep-frying, a dangerous method of food preparation. The dangers result from rapid oxidation and other chemical changes that take place when oils are subjected to high temperatures in the presence of light and oxygen. Some unhealthy trans-fatty acids result, as well as numerous other more toxic oxidation products. To avoid this, our falafels are baked, without sacrificing flavor or texture.

ANALYSIS FOR 1 SERVING:
2 balls with low-sodium soy sauce and 1 tablespoon Garlic Tahini Sauce

Calories: 217, Fat: 9.7 g, Total carbohydrates: 23.4 g, Protein: 12.4 g,
Dietary fiber: 6.1 g, Sodium: 455 mg, Net carbs: 17.3 g, Carb Choice: 1

ANALYSIS FOR 1 SERVING:
2 balls with low-sodium soy sauce

Calories: 154, Fat: 4.3 g, Total carbohydrates: 20.4 g, Protein: 10.5 g,
Dietary fiber: 5.1 g, Sodium: 354 mg, Net carbs: 15.3 g, Carb Choice: 1

ANALYSIS FOR 1 SERVING:
2 balls with Bragg Liquid Aminos

Calories: 154, Fat: 4.7 g, Total carbohydrates: 20.3 g, Protein: 10.9 g,
Dietary fiber: 5.4 g, Sodium: 418 mg, Net carbs: 14.9 g, Carb Choice: 1

Aunt Vienna's Mushroom and Black Bean Burger

Heavy on the fiber from the black beans and oats, this recipe makes a great hamburger alternative that's low-fat, low-calorie, and low-carb. It can also be served with a simple mushroom gravy as an entrée.

¼ cup (2 ounces) Mori-Nu lite, firm silken tofu

1 (4-ounce) can or jar mushroom stems and pieces, drained and coarsely chopped

½ cup unsweetened soymilk

1 small diced onion

¼ cup regular-sodium canned black beans, drained and slightly mashed with a fork

1 tablespoon McKay's Beef-Style Instant Broth and Seasoning, Vegan

5 tablespoons water

1 tablespoon low-sodium soy sauce

⅛ teaspoon cayenne pepper

¼ teaspoon seasoned salt

1¼ cups old-fashioned rolled oats

Cooking spray

■ In a small bowl, mash the tofu with a fork. Add the remaining ingredients except the oats, and mix together well. Add the oats, mix well, and let sit for 15 minutes to thicken. Spray a large skillet with cooking spray, and heat over medium heat. Measure patty-size portions of ⅓ or ½ cup, place patties in skillet, and press lightly with a spoon to flatten and shape. Cook for 5 minutes, spray patties for 2 seconds with cooking spray, turn, and cook for 5 minutes.

▶ *Nutrition Note:* See 10-Minute Burger (page 125) for more information on soy versus meat burgers and buns.

ANALYSIS FOR 1 SERVING:
⅓-cup patty

Calories: 68, Fat: 1.2 g, Total carbohydrates: 11.1 g, Protein: 3.6 g, Dietary fiber: 2.1 g, Sodium: 243 mg, Net carbs: 9.0 g, Carb Choice: ½

ANALYSIS FOR 1 SERVING:
½-cup patty

Calories: 101, Fat: 1.9 g, Total carbohydrates: 16.6 g, Protein: 5.4 g, Dietary fiber: 3.2 g, Sodium: 365 mg, Net carbs: 13.4 g, Carb Choice: 1

Black Bean Enchiladas

MAKES 6 ENCHILADAS; 6 SERVINGS

*W*hat could be better than soft corn tortillas tightly rolled with hearty black beans and fragrant cilantro, topped with a chili-laced sauce? Drizzle with our homemade Cashew Jack Cheese Sauce (page 213) and put the "olé!" back in your day. You may serve them with LCA Basic Tofu Sour Cream (page 220), Tofu Sour Cream Supreme (page 235), Low-Fat Tofu Sour Cream (page 224), Tofu Cilantro Sour Cream (page 233), or Tofutti Better Than Sour Cream. A plastic squirt bottle makes drizzling cheese sauce on these enchiladas easy and fun.

ENCHILADA SAUCE

1 (8-ounce) can tomato sauce (1 cup)

½ cup water

⅛ teaspoon ground cumin

3 tablespoons jarred salsa

1½ teaspoons chili powder

½ (12-ounce) bag Morningstar Farms Grillers Recipe Crumbles, thawed, or other meatless burger crumbles

1 teaspoon dry onion soup mix, nonhydrogenated

½ cup low-sodium canned black beans, drained

¼ cup finely chopped onion

2 tablespoons chopped fresh cilantro

½ cup Cashew Jack Cheese Sauce (page 213)

6 Food for Life Sprouted Corn tortillas

- **Make the sauce:** Stir all the sauce ingredients together in a saucepan, and simmer for 5 minutes.
- Mix all the ingredients together in a bowl, except the tortillas, enchilada sauce, and ¼ cup cheese sauce, and set aside.
- Preheat the oven to 350°F. To assemble, spread half of the Enchilada Sauce on the bottom of an 8-inch-square baking dish. Soften the tortillas before filling by briefly heating on both sides in a nonstick skillet over medium heat. Put ¼ cup of the filling in a tortilla, roll up, and place seam-side down in prepared baking dish. Repeat with remaining tortillas and filling. Drizzle remaining Enchilada Sauce down the center of the enchiladas, then top with remaining cheese sauce. Bake for 15 minutes, until the sauce is bubbly and the enchiladas are heated through.

ANALYSIS FOR 1 SERVING:
1 enchilada without toppings

Calories: 153, Fat: 2.8 g, Carbohydrates: 25.8 g, Protein: 7.7 g,
Dietary fiber: 4.1 g, Sodium: 552 mg, Net carbs: 21.7 g, Carb Choice: 1½

Chunky Chickpea Pita Pockets

MAKES 2 SERVINGS; ½ FILLED PITA EACH

Whenever guests leave our Sulphur, Oklahoma, or Sedona, Arizona, campuses (either for picnics or to head home), we have the chef pack them a few of these sandwiches to go, on Ezekiel 4:9 Prophet's pocket bread, complete with lettuce and tomato.

1 Ezekiel 4:9 Prophet's pocket bread or other whole wheat pita bread

⅔ cup Chunky Chickpea Spread (page 215)

⅔ cup finely chopped romaine or other dark green lettuce

4 tablespoons finely chopped tomato

■ Cut the pocket bread in half. Fill each half with ⅓ cup of the chickpea spread, and top with ⅓ cup of the lettuce and 2 tablespoons of the tomato.

> **ANALYSIS FOR 1 SERVING:**
> ½ filled pita pocket
>
> Calories: 167, Fat: 4.3 g, Total carbohydrates: 25.6 g, Protein: 8.4 g, Dietary fiber: 6.6 g, Sodium: 266 mg, Net carbs: 19 g, Carb Choice: 1

Crabby Cakes and No-Mayo Tartar Sauce

MAKES 4 (⅓-CUP) PATTIES; 4 SERVINGS

This quick and easy bean patty has a hearty, crunchy texture, and (we're told over and over again by LCA guests) a pleasantly fishlike flavor, especially when topped with No-Mayo Tartar Sauce (page 226).

1½ cups Chunky Chickpea Spread (page 215)

¼ cup garbanzo flour

1 teaspoon McKay's Chicken-Style Instant Broth and Seasoning, Vegan

Cooking spray

2 tablespoons plus 2 teaspoons No-Mayo Tartar Sauce (page 226)

■ Mix the chickpea spread with flour and seasoning. Measure ⅓-cup portions and form into patties. Spray a frying pan with cooking spray for 4 seconds and heat over medium heat. Add the patties and cook until crispy on the bottom. Spray each patty for 1 second, flip over, and cook until crispy. Top each patty with 2 teaspoons of the sauce.

ANALYSIS FOR 1 SERVING:
1 patty with 2 teaspoons No-Mayo Tartar Sauce

Calories: 153, Fat: 7.2 g, Total carbohydrates: 17.7 g, Protein: 5.6 g, Dietary fiber: 4.4 g, Sodium: 271 mg, Net carbs: 13.3 g, Carb Choice: 1

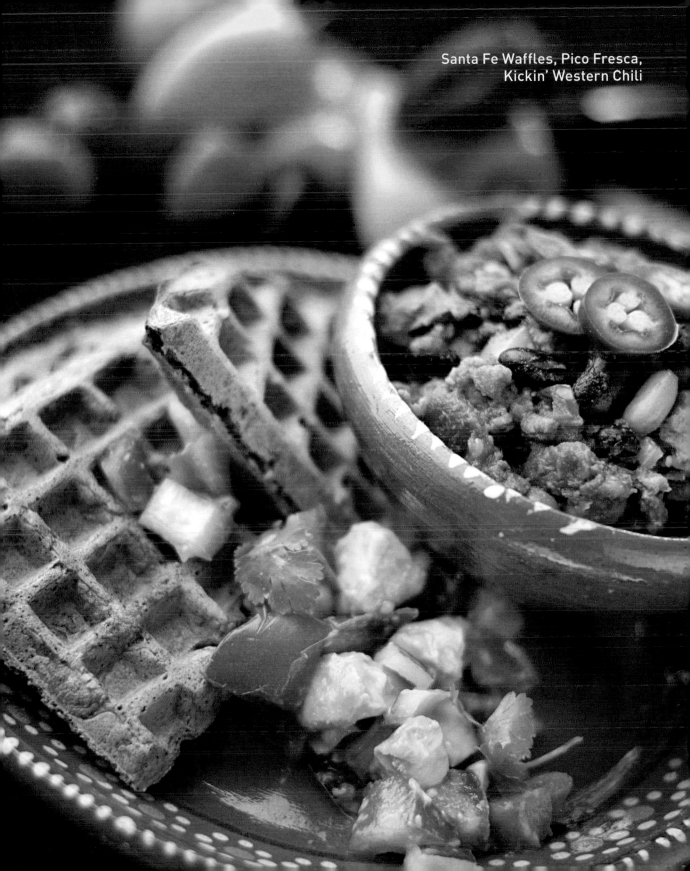

Santa Fe Waffles, Pico Fresca,
Kickin' Western Chili

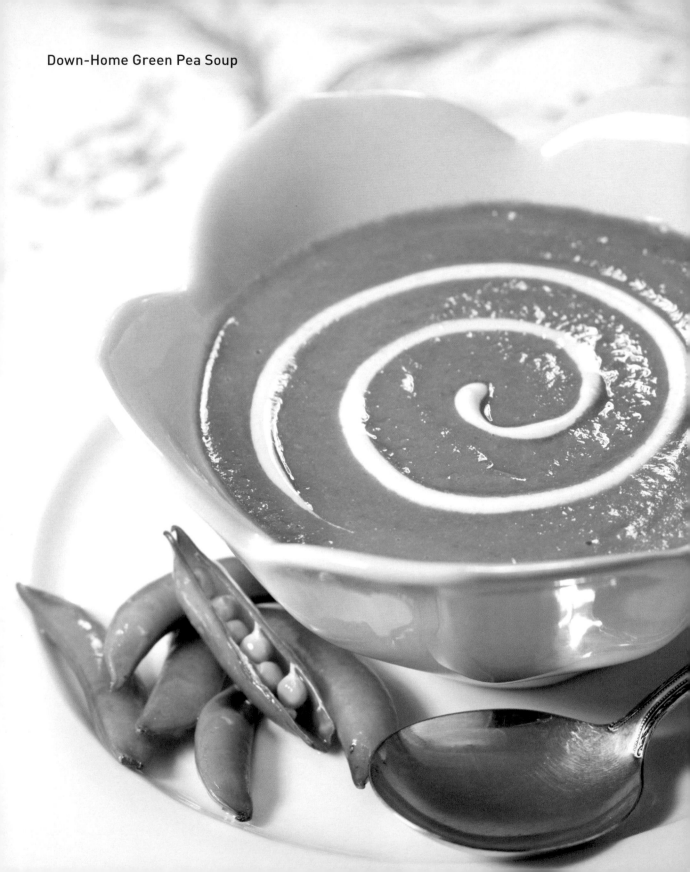

Down-Home Green Pea Soup

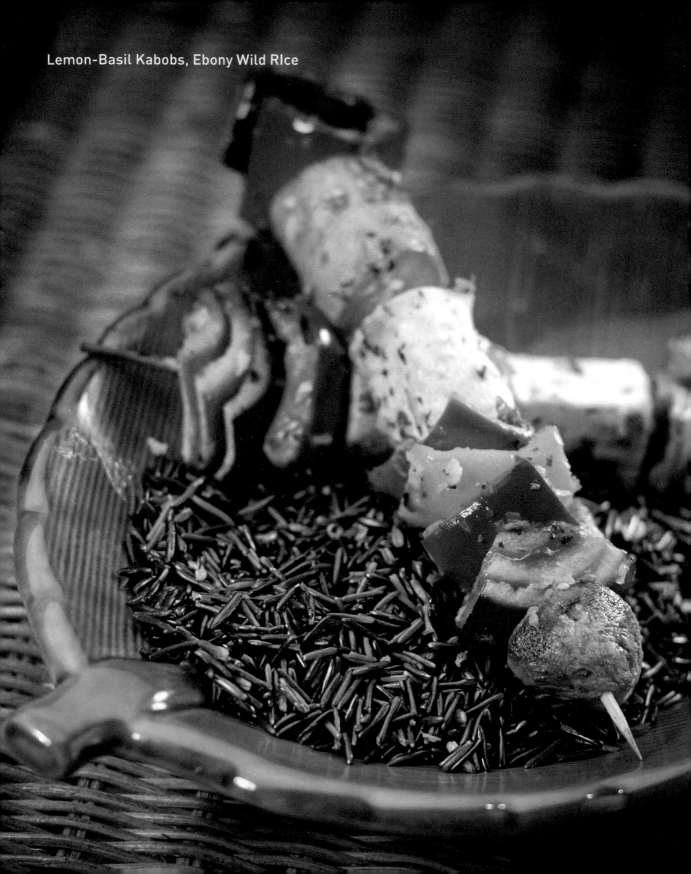

Lemon-Basil Kabobs, Ebony Wild RIce

Deluxe Lentil Soup

This country soup is very warming and so full of flavor and substance it works as a main dish. Snuggle up to a hot bowl on a chilly winter day.

½ cup brown lentils

4 cups water

1 tablespoon extra-virgin olive oil

1 garlic clove

1 cup chopped onion

½ cup diced celery

¾ cup sliced carrot

1½ cups ½-inch peeled red potato cubes

1½ teaspoons McKay's Beef Style Instant Broth and Seasoning, Vegan

1 teaspoon salt

1 teaspoon ground cumin

1 cup diced fresh tomatoes

¾ teaspoon seasoned salt

¼ teaspoon dried basil

¼ teaspoon ground coriander

¼ teaspoon sweet paprika

2 tablespoons chopped fresh parsley

■ Simmer the lentils and water in a pot, covered, for 1 hour. Heat the olive oil in a skillet over medium heat. Add the garlic and onion and sauté until tender, 3 to 4 minutes. Add to the lentils, along with the celery, carrot, potatoes, seasoning, salt, and cumin. Simmer, covered, until the potatoes are soft, about 15 minutes. Add the tomatoes, seasoned salt, basil, coriander, and paprika, and cook for 5 minutes. Garnish with the parsley and serve.

▶ *Nutrition Note:* Lentils have been a staple source of protein for millions of people in non-Western cultures for thousands of years. Like all dried beans, they are well-supplied with complex carbohydrates, fiber, and protein. They're a good source of thiamin, vitamin B_6, potassium, and zinc, and they're a particularly rich source of iron and the B vitamin folate. One-half cup of cooked lentils provides almost half the daily requirement of folate.

> **ANALYSIS FOR 1 SERVING:**
> 1 cup
>
> Calories: 100, Fat: 2.1 g, Total carbohydrates: 17.2 g, Protein: 4.3 g, Dietary fiber: 4.3 g, Sodium: 476 mg, Net carbs: 12.9 g, Carb Choice: 1

Gourmet Eggplant Stacks

Crisp on the outside, deliciously tender within, these eggplant slices make a stunning presentation when stacked and garnished with fresh basil.

1 large eggplant

½ cup Creamy Ranch Dressing (page 104) or Low-Fat Tofu Mayonnaise (page 223)

·2 cups Healthy Breading Mix (opposite)

2¼ cups Chunky Marinara Sauce (page 216)

1 cup Tofu Cottage Cheese (page 117)

⅔ cup Cashew Jack Cheese Sauce (page 213)

- Preheat the oven to 350°F. Spray a baking sheet with cooking spray. Wash eggplant and cut into 18 round slices. Lightly coat slices with ranch dressing and dip into breading mix. Place eggplant on prepared baking sheet, and bake for 10 minutes on each side to brown evenly. Leave oven on.
- **Assemble stacks:** Place a large piece of baked eggplant on another baking pan. Top with 2 tablespoons of the marinara sauce, followed by about 1¾ tablespoons of the Tofu Cottage Cheese. Place a smaller slice of baked eggplant on top, followed by 2 tablespoons of marinara sauce and about 1 tablespoon of the cheese sauce. Repeat until 9 two-tiered stacks are made. Bake again at 350°F for 10 to 15 minutes and serve immediately.

> *Nutrition Note:* See Nutrition Note for Succulent Ratatouille (page 160) to learn more about eggplant.

ANALYSIS FOR 1 SERVING:
1 stack

Calories: 145, Fat: 4.4 g, Total carbohydrates: 22.7 g, Protein: 6.5 g, Dietary fiber: 4.3 g, Sodium: 441 mg, Net carbs: 18.4 g, Carb Choice: 1

Healthy Breading Mix

MAKES 2 CUPS

This low-carb, whole grain breading mix can be used for our Quick and Easy Eggplant (page 156), Gourmet Eggplant Stacks (opposite), or to bread cauliflower or other vegetables. You can even use it as a vegetable stuffing. We use Ezekiel 4:9 Sprouted Grain bread because it's a whole grain bread that's flourless, and contains beans, making it more diabetic-friendly. You may use any whole grain bread as a substitute. You can also make this in a blender, adding 1 to 2 slices at a time.

5 slices Ezekiel 4:9 Sprouted Grain bread or other whole grain bread

½ teaspoon sweet paprika

½ teaspoon onion powder

¼ teaspoon garlic powder

1 teaspoon Italian seasoning

■ Tear the bread into pieces, put into a food processor, and process on medium into crumbs, 2 to 4 minutes. Add seasonings and stir together.

ANALYSIS FOR 1 SERVING:
3½ tablespoons

Calories: 45, Fat: 0.3 g, Total carbohydrates: 9.3 g, Protein: 1.8 g, Dietary fiber: 1.1, Sodium: 41 mg, Net carbs: 8.2 g, Carb Choice: ½

Grilled Portobello Mushrooms

*S*pray, *then bake, grill or roast—that's all there is to perfecting these meaty-flavored, crisp-on-the-outside, tender-in-the-middle mushrooms, which make an excellent sandwich or "steak" entrée.*

4 large portobello mushrooms (about 3 ounces each)

5½ tablespoons reduced-calorie Italian vinaigrette dressing, Marinade for Lemon-Basil Kabobs (page 145), or Aioli (page 210)

4 tablespoons Mustard Sauce (page 225)

■ Preheat a broiler or grill to medium-high heat. Cut off the stems and wash mushrooms thoroughly and pat dry. Marinate the mushrooms in the vinaigrette while the broiler is preheating, turning to ensure both sides are coated. Place on a baking sheet, gills side up, and broil until brown and softened, 4 to 5 minutes. Turn over and brush the marinade onto each mushroom top. Broil until brown and tender, 4 to 5 minutes. Top each mushroom with 1 tablespoon of the Mustard Sauce and serve hot.

ANALYSIS FOR 1 SERVING:
1 grilled mushroom with 1 tablespoon Mustard Sauce

Calories: 79, Fat: 5.6 g, Total carbohydrates: 6.0 g, Protein: 3.0 g,
Dietary fiber: 1.3 g, Sodium: 247 mg, Net carbs: 5.1 g, Carb Choice: ⅓

Grilled Quesadilla

Our quesadilla is shaped like a turnover made from a whole grain flour tortilla grilled to perfection. Here, healthy nondairy cheese and vegetables provide the filling.

It may be topped with salsa, guacamole, Low-Fat Tofu Sour Cream (page 224), Tofu Cilantro Sour Cream (page 233), or Tofutti Better Than Sour Cream.

1 Ezekiel 4:9 Sprouted Grain tortilla

Cooking spray

½ cup Refried Frijoles Negros (page 189)

1 ounce Vegan Gourmet cheddar cheese alternative, grated (about ¼ cup), or other nondairy (no casein) cheese alternative

2 tablespoons chopped onion

1 Roma tomato, chopped

■ Spray the tortilla for 1 second on each side. Grill on both sides in a dry skillet over medium heat until soft. Remove the tortilla from the skillet and spread with the beans, sprinkle with cheese, and top with onion and tomato. Fold the tortilla in half and return to the skillet, cooking until the cheese is melted and the tortilla is golden brown on both sides; flip once or twice during cooking. Serve immediately.

▶ *Nutrition Note:* The analysis amounts in this recipe are higher than for most recipes because, with a salad on the side, this is designed to be a complete meal.

ANALYSIS FOR 1 SERVING:
1 quesadilla with no toppings

Calories: 393, Fat: 14.1 g, Total carbohydrates: 56.9 g, Protein: 16.6 g,
Dietary fiber: 12.4 g, Sodium: 310 mg, Net carbs: 44.5 g, Carb Choice: 3

Haystacks

*O*ne *of the most popular meals at LCA, haystacks are fun, filling, and flexible, depending on what toppings you have around the kitchen. A haystack is a meal in itself, with no side dishes necessary. Any of our bean recipes work well when making Haystacks, and you can also substitute other vegetables.*

1 cup Kickin' Western Chili (page 143)

1 ounce (18 chips) Guiltless Gourmet Baked Yellow Corn tortilla chips or other low-fat, whole grain baked corn chips

1½ cups shredded lettuce

½ cup diced tomato

2 tablespoons diced onion

⅛ medium avocado, diced (about ⅛ cup)

1 tablespoon chopped or sliced black olives

Salsa Fresca (page 229), Chiapas Salsa (page 214), or other salsa (optional)

Soy sour cream (optional)

■ Heat the chili. Layer the ingredients on a plate in the following order: chips, chili, and vegetables. Top with salsas or soy sour cream (if using).

▶ *Nutrition Note:* The analysis amounts in this recipe are higher than for most recipes because this is designed to be a complete meal.

> **ANALYSIS FOR 1 SERVING:**
> 1 haystack without optional toppings
>
> Calories: 396, Fat: 9.7 g, Total carbohydrates: 63.8 g, Protein: 18.0 g,
> Dietary fiber: 15.5 g, Sodium: 740 mg, Net carbs: 48.3 g, Carb Choice: 3

Italian Stuffed Shells

Mama Mia! This easy make-ahead meal is perfect for entertaining. If you don't have time to make a homemade sauce, try Classico Roasted Garlic spaghetti sauce, which is low in sodium and very tasty. You can find whole grain giant pasta shells at your health food store, but if you can't find the giant variety, you can use any whole wheat pasta shell or whole wheat manicotti shell.

6 whole grain giant pasta shells

1¼ cups Chunky Marinara Sauce (page 216)

1½ cups Italian Tofu Filling (page 142)

■ Preheat the oven to 350°F. Cook the shells in unsalted water until al dente, rinse, and cool. Spread ½ cup of the marinara sauce evenly on the bottom of an 8-inch-square baking dish. Stuff each shell with ¼ cup of the filling, and place in the baking dish, open side up. Spoon 2 tablespoons of the remaining marinara sauce over each stuffed shell. Cover with foil or lid and bake for 15 minutes; uncover and bake for an additional 5 minutes.

ANALYSIS FOR 1 SERVING:
1 stuffed shell with Italian Tofu Filling using Tofutti sour cream

Calories: 124, Fat: 5.7 g, Total carbohydrates: 14.2 g, Protein: 6.7 g, Dietary fiber: 2.1 g, Sodium: 375 mg, Net carbs: 12.1 g, Carb Choice: ⅔

ANALYSIS FOR 1 SERVING:
1 stuffed shell with Italian Tofu Filling using Nayonaise spread

Calories: 121, Fat: 6.3 g, Total Carbohydrates: 11.9 g, Protein: 6.5 g, Dietary fiber: 1.9 g, Sodium: 398 mg, Net carbs: 10 g, Carb Choice: ⅔

Italian Tofu Filling

1 teaspoon extra-virgin olive oil

½ cup finely chopped onion

2 cloves garlic, minced

1 teaspoon dried basil

1 teaspoon Italian seasoning

1½ cups water-packed, extra-firm tofu, drained, rinsed, crumbled

1 teaspoon onion powder

½ teaspoon garlic powder

½ teaspoon salt

¼ cup Tofutti Better Than Sour Cream or Nayonaise spread

1 tablespoon fresh lemon juice

■ Heat the oil in a skillet over medium heat. Add the onion and garlic and sauté until tender, 3 to 4 minutes. Add the basil and Italian seasoning and sauté for 1 to 2 minutes, stirring constantly. Add the tofu to the skillet and cook, stirring occasionally, until the mixture looks dry. Remove the skillet from the heat. Stir in the remaining ingredients and mix well.

ANALYSIS FOR 1 SERVING:
¼ cup with Tofutti Better Than Sour Cream

Calories: 84, Fat: 5.1 g, Total carbohydrates: 6.2 g, Protein: 5.1 g, Dietary fiber: 0.9 g, Sodium: 256 mg, Net carbs: 5.3 g, Carb Choice: ⅓

ANALYSIS FOR 1 SERVING:
¼ cup with Nayonaise spread

Calories: 81, Fat: 5.8 g, Total carbohydrates: 3.8 g, Protein: 5.0 g, Dietary fiber: 0.7 g, Sodium: 278 mg, Net carbs: 3.1 g, Carb Choice: free

---

Kickin' Western Chili

MAKES 9 CUPS; 18 (½-CUP) SERVINGS WITH BURGER CRUMBLES
MAKES 7 CUPS; 14 (½-CUP) SERVINGS WITHOUT BURGER CRUMBLES

This first-place chili cook-off winner is bursting with fabulous textures and flavors. The longer it cooks, the better it gets. At Windcrest Restaurant, we serve these beans every day— for breakfast! We know this is a large batch of chili. Divide leftover chili into portions that fit your needs, and freeze. Thaw in the microwave or overnight in the refrigerator.

1½ teaspoons extra-virgin olive oil

1½ cups chopped onions

¼ cup chopped green bell pepper

3 cloves garlic, minced

2 tablespoons chili powder, or to taste

1½ teaspoons ground cumin

⅛ teaspoon dried oregano

¾ teaspoon sweet paprika

3 cups Morningstar Farms Grillers Recipe Crumbles, thawed, or other meatless burger crumbles (optional)

1 (15-ounce) can regular-sodium canned pinto beans, drained (1½ cups)

1 (15-ounce) can regular-sodium canned red kidney beans, drained (1½ cups)

1 (15-ounce) can regular-sodium canned black beans, drained (1½ cups)

1 (14.5-ounce) can diced tomatoes (1½ cups)

¼ cup tomato paste

2 tablespoons canned chopped mild green chilies

1½ cups water

■ Heat the oil in a large saucepan over medium heat. Add the onions, bell pepper, and garlic, and sauté until tender, 4 to 5 minutes. Stir in the seasonings and crumbles (if using), and sauté for 1 minute. Add the remaining ingredients, bring to a boil, reduce the heat, and simmer until the flavors are blended, 30 to 45 minutes.

▶ *Nutrition Note:* To lower the sodium in this recipe, use low-sodium canned beans.

ANALYSIS FOR 1 SERVING:
½ cup with burger crumbles

Calories: 97, Fat: 1.5 g, Total carbohydrates: 15.8 g, Protein: 6.4 g, Dietary fiber: 4.5 g, Sodium: 238 mg, Net carbs: 11.3 g, Carb Choice: ⅔

ANALYSIS FOR 1 SERVING:
½ cup without burger crumbles

Calories: 101, Fat: 1.1 g, Total carbohydrates: 18.6 g, Protein: 5.6 g, Dietary fiber: 5.2 g, Sodium: 281 mg, Net carbs: 13.4 g, Carb Choice: 1

Lemon-Basil Kabobs

MAKES 12 KABOBS; 6 (2-KABOB) SERVINGS

Thick chunks of vegetables and tofu are marinated in a tangy sauce, then baked on a wooden skewer. Serve with our Ebony Wild Rice (page 193) and a leafy green salad, and you have a scrumptious plant-based meal for a summer gathering of family and friends.

2 large carrots, cut into 1-inch wedges

1 medium red onion, cut into 12 (2-inch) squares

1 large green bell pepper, cut into 1-inch squares

1 large red bell pepper, cut into 1-inch squares

12 medium button mushrooms

3 Roma tomatoes, quartered, seeds removed

1 large zucchini, cut into 1¼-inch slices

1 large sweet potato, peeled, cut into 1-inch cubes

2 cups package water-packed, extra-firm tofu, drained, cut into 12 (1 × 1½-inch) chunks

1 recipe Marinade for Lemon-Basil Kabobs (opposite)

■ Assemble the kabobs, alternating ingredients, and place in a large glass baking dish. Pour the marinade over the kabobs, cover, and marinate overnight in the refrigerator.

■ Preheat the oven to 400°F. Spray a baking sheet with cooking spray. Place the kabobs on prepared baking sheet, and bake for 12 to 15 minutes. Serve immediately.

ANALYSIS FOR 1 SERVING:
2 kabobs without marinade

Calories: 153, Fat: 4.2 g, Total carbohydrates: 23.1 g, Protein: 9.8 g, Dietary fiber: 5.5 g, Sodium: 25 mg, Net carbs: 17.6 g, Carb Choice: 1

ANALYSIS FOR 1 SERVING:
2 kabobs with 1 tablespoon marinade

Calories: 202, Fat: 9.0 g, Total carbohydrates: 24.6 g, Protein: 10.4 g, Dietary fiber: 5.8 g, Sodium: 239 mg, Net carbs: 18.8 g, Carb Choice: 1

Marinade for Lemon-Basil Kabobs

*M*ost marinades are heavy on the oil, and therefore high-calorie and high-fat. This one is flavorful, but low on fat and calories. It can also be used for Grilled Portobello Mushrooms (page 138) or any other grilled vegetable.

3 cups coarsely chopped onions
¾ cup canola oil
½ cup Bragg Liquid Aminos

1 cup fresh lemon juice
1 tablespoon dried basil
1 teaspoon salt

■ Pulse the onions in a blender on high until they turn to liquid, about 1 minute. Add the remaining ingredients and blend until creamy, about 15 seconds.

> **ANALYSIS FOR 1 SERVING:**
> 1 tablespoon
>
> Calories: 25, Fat: 2.4 g, Total carbohydrates: 0.8 g, Protein: 0.3 g,
> Dietary fiber: 0.2 g, Sodium: 107 mg, Net carbs: 0.6 g, Carb Choice: free

Linda B.'s Sesame Lettuce Wraps with Thai Peanut Sauce

MAKES 2 CUPS; 8 (¼-CUP) SERVINGS

This dish features tofu grilled in fragrant sesame oil and drizzled with a mildly sweet peanut sauce. Serve warm in a crisp lettuce leaf for a delightful Asian side dish or appetizer. Known for its long, sturdy leaves, romaine lettuce works well for this wrap, though many people prefer the crispness of an iceberg leaf.

½ teaspoon canola oil

2¼ teaspoons toasted sesame oil

¼ cup finely chopped onion

3 green onions, minced

1 clove garlic, minced

2 tablespoons grated carrot

1¼ cups drained water-packed, extra-firm tofu, cut into ¼-inch cubes

¼ cup Morningstar Farms Grillers Recipe Crumbles, thawed, or other meatless burger crumbles

1 tablespoon low-sodium soy sauce

1½ teaspoons McKay's Chicken-Style Instant Broth and Seasoning, Vegan

1 tablespoon 100 percent natural floral honey

Pinch cayenne pepper (optional)

8 large lettuce leaves

8 tablespoons Thai Peanut Sauce (page 232)

■ Heat the oils in a skillet over medium heat. Add the chopped onion, green onions, garlic, carrot, tofu cubes, and crumbles, and sauté until the onion is tender, 3 to 4 minutes. Stir in the remaining ingredients, except the lettuce and sauce, and cook for 4 to 5 minutes to blend the flavors. Remove from the heat and allow to cool briefly before using. Place ¼ cup in each lettuce leaf, drizzle with 1 tablespoon of the sauce, and roll like a burrito. Fasten each lettuce leaf with a wooden pick if arranging on a platter.

> **ANALYSIS FOR 1 SERVING:**
> 1 filled lettuce leaf with 1 tablespoon Thai Peanut Sauce
>
> Calories: 123, Fat: 8.2 g, Total carbohydrates: 8.0 g, Protein: 6.8 g,
> Dietary fiber: 1.2 g, Sodium: 178 mg, Net carbs: 6.8 g, Carb Choice: ½

Mazidra

*L*entils are inexpensive, nutritious, and quick to cook. Mazidra is a traditional Mediterranean dish consisting of brown rice smothered in these healthy little high-fiber jewels, and topped with lettuce, tomatoes, and onions and served with a side of steamed veggies. We serve ours over Mellow Brown Rice (page 194) or Ebony Wild Rice (page 193), topped with shredded lettuce, chopped tomato, diced onion, and our delicious Low-Fat Tofu Sour Cream (page 224).

1 tablespoon extra-virgin olive oil
½ cup chopped onion
3 cloves garlic, minced
3 cups water
1 cup dry lentils
½ teaspoon dried basil

½ teaspoon dried oregano
2 bay leaves
2 teaspoons McKay's Beef-Style Instant Broth and Seasoning, Vegan
1 (8-ounce) can tomato sauce (1 cup)
¾ cup canned diced tomatoes
½ teaspoon salt

■ Heat the olive oil in a large saucepan over medium heat. Add the onion and garlic and sauté until tender, 3 to 4 minutes. Add the water, lentils, basil, oregano, bay leaves, and beef-style seasoning. Cover and cook until the lentils are soft, 40 to 50 minutes. Add the tomato sauce, tomatoes, and salt, and bring to a boil. Remove the bay leaves and serve immediately.

ANALYSIS FOR 1 SERVING:
¾ cup cooked lentils without rice or toppings

Calories: 135, Fat: 2.5 g, Total carbohydrates: 21.6 g, Protein: 8.2 g,
Dietary fiber: 7.3 g, Sodium: 461 mg. Net carbs: 14.3 g, Carb Choice: 1

Nut Meatballs

Here's a healthy version of an Italian classic. Pecans add bulk, flavor, and texture. Our Chunky Marinara Sauce (page 216) with its hints of basil and garlic is the perfect partner to these savory meatballs and whole grain pasta. For extra flavor, use Toasted Pecans (page 207).

1½ cups Morningstar Farms Grillers Recipe Crumbles, thawed, or other meatless burger crumbles

1½ teaspoons Bragg Liquid Aminos

1½ teaspoons extra-virgin olive oil

¼ cup chopped onion

¼ teaspoon garlic powder

⅛ teaspoon dried basil

½ teaspoon McKay's Beef-Style Instant Broth and Seasoning, Vegan

2 tablespoons gluten flour

2 tablespoons plus 2 teaspoons whole wheat flour

1½ teaspoons Red Star nutritional yeast flakes

2 tablespoons finely chopped pecans, walnuts, or almonds

Pinch sweet paprika

■ Preheat the oven to 350°F. Spray a large baking pan with cooking spray. Marinate the crumbles in the Bragg Liquid Aminos and oil for 10 minutes. Add the remaining ingredients and mix together well. Divide into 2-tablespoon portions and shape into balls. Place in prepared baking pan, and cover with foil. Bake for 15 minutes; uncover, and bake for 5 minutes. Meatballs are done when firm yet springy.

ANALYSIS FOR 1 SERVING:
2 balls with no sauce, made with pecans

Calories: 97, Fat: 3.8 g, Total carbohydrates: 6.5 g, Protein: 10.1 g, Dietary fiber: 1.7 g, Sodium: 124 mg, Net carbs: 4.8 g, Carb Choice: ⅓

Party Pasta Bake

This is a one-dish meal ideal for a buffet, or meant to be made ahead and reheated when there's no time for cooking. It's also perfect for potlucks. Don't rinse your pasta after cooking. Sticky pasta helps bind this dish together.

6 ounces whole grain macaroni or similar small pasta (1¼ cups)

½ cup chopped yellow onion

2 cloves garlic, minced

2 tablespoons water

1 cup Morningstar Farms Grillers Recipe Crumbles, thawed, or other meatless burger crumbles

1 teaspoon Italian seasoning

2 teaspoons dried basil

1¾ cups Classico Roasted Garlic spaghetti sauce

½ (14.5-ounce) can low-sodium tomatoes, half of liquid reserved

½ medium zucchini, cut into ¾-inch cubes (about 1¼ cups)

2 tablespoons chopped fresh parsley, plus additional fresh parsley for garnish (optional), or 1½ teaspoons dried parsley

¾ cup Tofu Cottage Cheese (page 117) or Italian Tofu Filling (page 142)

1/16 teaspoon cayenne pepper, or to taste

2 ounces Vegan Gourmet mozzarella cheese alternative or other nondairy (no casein) cheese alternative, grated (8 tablespoons)

- Preheat the oven to 350°F. Spray an 8-inch-square baking dish with cooking spray. Cook the pasta in plain boiling water (no oil or salt added), until al dente. Drain and set aside.
- Sauté the onion and garlic in the 2 tablespoons water until tender, 3 to 4 minutes. Add the crumbles and sauté for 1 to 2 minutes. Add the Italian seasoning and ½ teaspoon of the basil, and sauté for 1 to 2 minutes. Stir in the spaghetti sauce, tomatoes, zucchini, and parsley, and let simmer for 15 to 20 minutes.
- While the sauce is simmering, combine the Tofu Cottage Cheese, cayenne, and the remaining 1½ teaspoons basil. Mix in 6 tablespoons of the cheese alternative. Set aside.
- **Assemble the casserole:** Place the cooked pasta in the baking dish, add two-thirds of the sauce to the pasta, and mix well. Spread the cheese mixture evenly over the pasta. Top with the remaining sauce.
- Bake for 20 minutes. Sprinkle with the remaining 2 tablespoons cheese alternative and bake for 10 minutes, until bubbly. Garnish with parsley (if using).

Nut Butter Pâté

The mild taste of peanuts and a consistency somewhere between meatloaf and traditional pâté, makes this unusual dish a winner with kids and adults. You can enjoy this salty-sweet, low-carb nut loaf either warm or cold, plain, or sliced on a sandwich with soy mayonnaise and some lettuce and tomato. And yes, the unusual oven temperature for baking is correct. If possible, use ½ of an Ezekiel 4:9 Sprouted Grain bun, and 1 slice of 100 percent whole wheat bread. Place in a dry food processor to make quick crumbs. Spread crumbs on an unsprayed baking sheet or toaster oven pan, and dry in a 315°F oven for 7 minutes. Measure 1 cup of dry crumbs for this recipe.

1 cup no-salt-added canned tomatoes with juice, whole or diced

2 tablespoons creamy, all-natural, no-sugar-added, nonhydrogenated peanut butter with salt

⅓ cup chopped onion

1 cup dry bread crumbs from Ezekiel 4:9 Sprouted Grains burger buns or other whole grain bread

¾ teaspoon salt

½ teaspoon dried sage

■ Preheat the oven to 315°F. Spray an 8 × 4-inch loaf pan with cooking spray. Blend the tomatoes, peanut butter, and onion in a blender on high until smooth and creamy, about 1 minute. Pour blended mixture into a bowl and add the bread crumbs, salt, and sage, and stir together. Pour mixture into prepared pan. Gently shake the pan to level the loaf. Bake uncovered for 1½ hours, until the loaf is set and slightly pulled away from the edges of the pan. Cool completely before slicing, and warm in microwave for 30 seconds before eating, if desired.

ANALYSIS FOR 1 SERVING:
1-inch slice

Calories: 70, Fat: 2.8 g, Total carbohydrates: 9.6 g, Protein: 2.8 g, Dietary fiber: 1.6 g, Sodium: 323 mg, Net carbs: 8.0 g, Carb Choice: ½

Pasta e Fagioli

Basil, one of our favorite herbs, is one of the important flavors in this traditional Italian soup. Served with a green salad and our Southern Country Cornbread (page 180) or a slice of Sprouted Grain bread, this soup is a meal in itself. Regularly check the freshness of your dried herbs. They should be kept no longer than 6 to 9 months unless frozen.

2 tablespoons Smart Balance Light Buttery Spread

1 teaspoon extra-virgin olive oil

2 cups chopped onions

4 cloves garlic, minced

1 teaspoon dried basil

½ teaspoon Italian seasoning

2½ cups regular-sodium canned Great Northern beans, drained

3 cups water

2 tablespoons McKay's Chicken-Style Instant Broth and Seasoning, Vegan

1¼ cups low-sodium canned diced tomatoes with liquid

¹⁄₁₆ teaspoon cayenne pepper

½ teaspoon salt

2 bay leaves

¼–½ teaspoon dried rosemary (optional)

1 cup whole grain macaroni

■ Heat the spread and olive oil in a large saucepan over medium heat. Add the onions and garlic and sauté until the onions are tender, 3 to 4 minutes. Add the basil and Italian seasoning and sauté for 1 minute. Stir in the remaining ingredients, except the pasta. Bring to a boil and simmer, uncovered, for about 10 minutes. Stir in the pasta and cook until tender, about 15 minutes. Remove the bay leaves and serve.

ANALYSIS FOR 1 SERVING:
1 cup

Calories: 207, Fat: 3.4 g, Total carbohydrates: 36.2 g, Protein: 10.3 g, Dietary fiber: 7.4 g, Sodium: 291 mg, Net carbs: 28.8 g, Carb Choice: 2

Pita Pizza with Alfredo Sauce

*T*hink pizza and good health can't coexist? Try our whole wheat, nondairy individual pizzas, and you'll be in for a surprise. These pizzas are loaded with chunky vegetarian toppings, so they're high in good vegetable protein and fiber, and much lower in fat than traditional pizza. Make all three varieties and serve them at your next party—nobody will miss the meat and cheese. The white bean and cashew Alfredo Sauce in this one gives it a tang that lends it more sophistication than the usual pizza. For a totally different flavor, substitute our Sun-Dried Tomato Dip (page 231) for the Alfredo Sauce.

3 tablespoons Alfredo Sauce (page 211)
1 Ezekiel 4:9 Prophet's pocket bread or other whole-wheat pita bread
¾ cup baby spinach leaves
1 medium Roma tomato, cut into 6 slices

1 tablespoon diced onion
¼ medium red bell pepper, cut into strips
1 teaspoon minced garlic
½ cup sliced mushrooms
Cooking spray

■ Preheat the oven to 400°F. Spread the Alfredo Sauce on top of the pita. In a small bowl, combine the spinach, tomato, onion, pepper, garlic, and mushrooms. Spray for 1 second with cooking spray and toss the vegetables together several times. Top the Alfredo Sauce with the vegetables. Place the pita on an unsprayed baking sheet and bake for about 12 minutes, until the vegetables are cooked al dente.

ANALYSIS FOR 1 SERVING:
1 pita pizza

Calories: 223, Fat: 5.7 g, Total carbohydrates: 34.3 g, Protein: 13.2 g,
Dietary fiber: 8.1 g, Sodium: 332 mg, Net carbs: 26.2 g, Carb Choice: 1⅔

Pita Pizza with Low-Fat Lifestyle Hummus

MAKES 1 PITA PIZZA; 1 SERVING

The hummus spread on this pizza provides a unique Middle Eastern flair to the traditional Italian-American favorite. For a totally different flavor, you can substitute our Aioli (page 210) for the Low-Fat Lifestyle Hummus in this recipe.

2 tablespoons dry sun-dried tomato strips

2 cloves garlic, peeled

Cooking spray

3 tablespoons Low-Fat Lifestyle Hummus (page 222)

1 Ezekiel 4:9 Prophet's pocket bread or other whole wheat pita

2 tablespoons diced red onion

1 canned artichoke heart, sliced

1 tablespoon diced green bell pepper

■ Rehydrate the sun-dried tomato by soaking in boiling water for about 1 hour.

■ Preheat the oven to 400°F. Spray the garlic with cooking spray, and roast in foil for 12 minutes. Spread the hummus on top of the pita. Drain the sun-dried tomato and sprinkle on the hummus along with the onion, artichoke heart, and pepper. Slice the roasted garlic and sprinkle on top of the vegetables. Place the pita on an unsprayed baking sheet and bake for 12 minutes, until the vegetables are cooked al dente.

ANALYSIS FOR 1 SERVING:
1 pita pizza

Calories: 240, Fat: 4.1 g, Total carbohydrates: 41.7 g, Protein: 13.2 g, Dietary fiber: 9.9 g, Sodium: 431 mg, Net carbs: 31.8 g, Carb Choice: 2

Pita Pizza with Refried Frijoles Negros

This pizza's a novel synthesis of Mexican and Italian-American favorites, with a medley of raw, fresh toppings kids will love.

3 tablespoons Refried Frijoles Negros (page 189)

1 Ezekiel 4:9 Prophet's pocket bread or other whole wheat pita

¾ cup finely shredded dark leaf lettuce

¼ cup diced fresh tomato

1 tablespoon diced red onion

2 tablespoons Pimiento Cheese Sauce (page 228) or 1 ounce Vegan Gourmet mozzarella cheese alternative or other nondairy (no casein) cheese alternative

■ Preheat the oven to 400°F. Spread the Refried Frijoles Negros on top of the pita. Place on an unsprayed baking sheet, and bake for 12 minutes, until fully heated and the bread crisps. Remove from the oven and top with the lettuce, tomato, onion, and sauce.

> **ANALYSIS FOR 1 SERVING:**
> 1 pita pizza with Pimiento Cheese Sauce
>
> Calories: 222, Fat: 3.9 g, Total carbohydrates: 37.2 g, Protein: 13.4 g, Dietary fiber: 9.1 g, Sodium: 296 mg, Net carbs: 28.1 g, Carb Choice: 2

Quick and Easy Eggplant

*M*ade *from one of our favorite summer vegetables, this is an easier version of our Gourmet Eggplant Stacks (page 136). Eggplant has a wonderfully meaty texture that works well in plant-based dishes as a substitute for meat. However, exercise caution when preparing eggplant: Even though it's almost a fat-free vegetable, it has an uncanny ability to rapidly absorb lots of fat. Don't fry or deep-fry it or use fat-rich mayonnaise or sour cream before breading it. See Nutrition Note for Succulent Ratatouille (page 160) to learn more about eggplant.*

1 large eggplant
½ cup Nayonaise spread
2 cups Healthy Breading Mix (page 137)

2¼ cups Chunky Marinara Sauce (page 216) or Classico Roasted Garlic spaghetti sauce

- Preheat the oven to 350°F. Spray a baking sheet with cooking spray. Wash, peel, and slice the eggplant into ½-inch-thick circles. Lightly coat both sides of each slice with Nayonaise and dip into the breading mix. Place breaded slices on prepared baking sheet, and bake for 10 minutes. Turn slices over and bake for another 10 minutes to brown evenly.
- Meanwhile, heat the sauce in a saucepan. Arrange eggplant stacks, two slices per stack, on a plate or in a serving dish. Top each stack with ¼ cup of the sauce.

ANALYSIS FOR 1 SERVING:
1 stack with ¼ cup Chunky Marinara Sauce

Calories: 122, Fat: 4.4 g, Total carbohydrates: 19.5 g, Protein: 3.4 g,
Dietary fiber: 3.8 g, Sodium: 324 mg, Net carbs: 15.7 g, Carb Choice: 1

ANALYSIS FOR 1 SERVING:
1 stack with ¼ cup Classico Roasted Garlic spaghetti sauce

Calories: 161, Fat: 5.8 g, Total carbohydrates: 26.7 g, Protein: 3.5 g,
Dietary fiber: 3.9 g, Sodium: 453 mg, Net carbs: 22.8 g, Carb Choice: 1½

Savory Dinner Roast

This main attraction is perfect for a potluck. We also like to serve it at holiday meals, nestled next to Smashed Potatoes (page 201) and gravy. Its meaty texture and flavor makes it especially welcome by people transitioning to a plant-based diet. It's also surprisingly low-calorie. Leftovers freeze well. This dish can also be sliced and served as a tasty sandwich with lettuce, tomatoes, and your favorite soy mayo.

2 cups water-packed, extra-firm tofu, drained

1 cup Morningstar Farms Grillers Recipe Crumbles, thawed, or other meatless burger crumbles

¼ cup chopped pecans

½ cup chopped onion

½ cup sliced black olives

¾ cup Cashew Jack Cheese Sauce (page 213)

¼ cup dry onion soup mix, nonhydrogenated

1 teaspoon garlic and herb seasoning (salt-free)

2 tablespoons Ener-G Egg Replacer

¼ cup water

2 teaspoons extra-virgin olive oil

4 cups organic Arrowhead Mills kamut flakes or other whole grain flaked cold cereal

■ Preheat the oven to 350°F. Spray a 13 × 9-inch baking dish with cooking spray. Rinse, drain, and mash the tofu in a medium bowl. Add the remaining ingredients, except the kamut flakes, and mix well. Fold in the kamut flakes and gently spread in prepared dish. Cover and bake for 20 minutes. Uncover and bake for 10 to 15 minutes, until firm in the middle and the top is browned.

ANALYSIS FOR 1 SERVING:
¹⁄₁₆ of 13 × 9-inch baking dish

Calories: 117, Fat: 5.6 g, Total carbohydrates: 12.0 g, Protein: 6.4 g, Dietary fiber: 1.8 g, Sodium: 279 mg, Net carbs: 10.2 g, Carb Choice: ⅔

Sombrero Olé

This is the perfect main course for a hot summer day, and it also makes a filling breakfast that's out of the ordinary. For a dramatic presentation, serve in our crispy oven-baked tortilla basket piled high with your favorite salsa and toppings.

1 Ezekiel 4:9 Sprouted Grain tortilla

Cooking spray

½ cup Refried Pinto Beans (page 190) or beans of your choice

1 cup shredded romaine lettuce

¼ cup chopped fresh tomato

2 tablespoons chopped onion

1 tablespoon chopped fresh cilantro

1 tablespoon Guacamole Rico (page 219)

■ Preheat the oven to 350°F. Spray one side of the tortilla with cooking spray for 2 seconds. Press sprayed side up in a 6-inch ovenproof bowl. Place a ball of foil in the bowl to hold the tortilla in place. Bake for 7 minutes, until the shell is crispy. Cool. Starting with the beans, fill with all the ingredients, and enjoy.

ANALYSIS FOR 1 SERVING:
1 Sombrero Olé

Calories: 335, Fat: 8.5 g, Total carbohydrates: 54.6 g, Protein: 15.4 g,
Dietary fiber: 13.4 g, Sodium: 431 mg, Net carbs: 41.2 g, Carb Choice: 2⅔

Spinach Lasagne

A make-ahead meal that is sure to please. Fresh spinach and the goodness of soy are layered between whole grain noodles and our tangy Chunky Marinara Sauce (page 216). Leftovers can actually taste better heated up the next day or two.

14 whole grain lasagne noodles

4 cups water-packed, extra-firm tofu, drained

½ cup unsweetened soymilk

2 teaspoons fresh lemon juice

1 cup finely chopped onion

8 cloves garlic, minced

4 cups chopped fresh spinach

2 tablespoons dried basil leaves

2 teaspoons dried oregano leaves

2 tablespoons Red Star nutritional yeast flakes

1½ teaspoons salt

5 cups Chunky Marinara Sauce (page 216)

■ Cook the noodles in plain boiling water (no oil or salt added), until al dente. Drain, pat dry with a paper towel, and set aside.

■ Preheat the oven to 350°F. Spray the bottom of a 13 × 9-inch baking dish with cooking spray. Process the tofu, soymilk, and lemon juice in a food processor until smooth. Spray a skillet with cooking spray. Add the onion, garlic, and spinach, and cook for 3 to 4 minutes. Fold the spinach mixture, basil, oregano, yeast flakes, and salt into the tofu filling mixture.

■ Spoon 1 cup of the marinara sauce over bottom of prepared dish. Lay 4 whole noodles lengthwise in the dish, and cut one to fill the remaining space. Spread the noodles with 3 cups of the filling mixture. Top the filling with another layer of noodles. Spread another 2 cups of the marinara sauce over the noodles. Spread another 3 cups of the filling over the sauce. Top with the remaining noodles and remaining 2 cups of sauce. Bake for 45 minutes, until the sauce bubbles. Allow to set for 10 minutes before cutting.

ANALYSIS FOR 1 SERVING:
1/16 of a 13 × 9-inch baking dish

Calories: 176, Fat: 5.6 g, Total carbohydrates: 23.2 g, Protein: 12.3 g, Dietary fiber: 3.5 g, Sodium: 467 mg, Net carbs: 19.7 g, Carb Choice: 1⅓

Succulent Ratatouille

This low-calorie, low-carb, high-fiber colorful stew features a captivating blend of herbs from the south of France. If you don't have herbes de Provence on hand, mix equal amounts of basil, marjoram, savory, and thyme, and add a pinch of rosemary.

2 tablespoons extra-virgin olive oil

1 cup yellow onion, cut into half-moons

3 cups ¾-inch unpeeled eggplant cubes

4 cups ¾-inch zucchini cubes

½ cup ⅜-inch green bell pepper squares

1 teaspoon salt

3 tablespoons water

¼ cup canned tomato puree

¾ teaspoon dried basil

1½ teaspoons herbes de Provence

2 cloves garlic, minced

3 cups ¾-inch fresh tomato cubes

■ Heat the olive oil in a large skillet over medium heat. Add the onion and eggplant and sauté, stirring often, until the eggplant is slightly browned and tender on the outside, about 10 minutes. Add the remaining ingredients, except the garlic and tomatoes, cover, and simmer, stirring occasionally, until the zucchini is half done, about 30 minutes. Add the garlic, cover, and simmer until the zucchini and eggplant are tender, 10 to 15 minutes. Add the tomatoes and cook until soft, 3 to 5 minutes.

▶ *Nutrition Note:* Eggplant is just about fat-free, with no noteworthy amounts of vitamins, phytochemicals, or minerals (except for potassium). To add insult to injury, the deep-purple phytochemical pigment in the skin is only on the outside of the eggplant, and that tends to get peeled off. However, eggplant is high in fiber, especially a respectable amount of cholesterol-lowering pectin. And eggplants do contain a class of phytochemicals known as saponins, which research suggests have antioxidant, anti-inflammatory, and cholesterol-lowering properties. Those same saponins are what give eggplant a bitter taste, which is alleviated when eggplant is cooked. However, don't salt the eggplant to get rid of the bitter taste or you will neutralize the beneficial saponins.

ANALYSIS FOR 1 SERVING:
1 cup

Calories: 98, Fat: 5.1 g, Total carbohydrates: 13.1 g, Protein: 2.7 g,
Dietary fiber: 3.9 g, Sodium: 447 mg, Net carbs: 9.2 g, Carb Choice: ⅔

Tex-Mex Casserole

This flavorful casserole is a spicy twist to lasagne, featuring layers of whole-grain corn tortillas, refried beans, and a nourishing green chili–tofu filling. Top with our Pimiento Cheese Sauce (page 228) to make a family favorite. If you really want an elegant presentation, instead of using the tortillas you can scoop this casserole into corn husks, which you can buy in the Mexican section of your grocery store. That's the way we serve this dish at Windcrest Restaurant.

1 cup plus 2 tablespoons jarred salsa

6 Food for Life Sprouted Corn tortillas or other 6-inch corn tortillas

2 cups Refried Pinto Beans (page 190)

2 cups Spicy Tofu Filling (recipe below)

■ Preheat the oven to 350°F. Lightly spray an 8-inch-square baking dish with cooking spray. Layer the ingredients in the baking dish in the following order: 6 tablespoons salsa, 2 corn tortillas, 1 cup beans, 1 cup filling. Repeat, ending with the remaining 6 tablespoons salsa. Cover with foil and bake for 30 minutes. Uncover and bake for 10 minutes, until the filling is set. Remove from the oven and let sit for 10 minutes. Cut into 8 portions.

ANALYSIS FOR 1 SERVING:
⅛ of an 8-inch-square baking dish

Calories: 183, Fat: 5.1 g, Total carbohydrates: 27.5 g, Protein: 9.3 g,
Dietary fiber: 6.0 g, Sodium: 551 mg, Net carbs: 21.5 g, Carb Choice: 1½

Spicy Tofu Filling

MAKES 2¾ CUPS

2 cups mashed, drained, water-packed, extra-firm tofu

¾ teaspoon salt

1¾ teaspoons onion powder

½ teaspoon garlic powder

1 tablespoon Red Star nutritional yeast flakes

½ cup plus 2 tablespoons Tofu Sour Cream Supreme (page 235) or Tofutti Better Than Sour Cream

⅛ teaspoon chili powder

¼ cup canned chopped mild green chilies

■ In a large bowl, combine all the ingredients and mix well. Cover and refrigerate until chilled.

ANALYSIS FOR 1 SERVING:
½ cup made with Tofu Sour Cream Supreme

Calories: 124, Fat: 7.8 g, Total carbohydrates: 7.4 g, Protein: 8.7 g,
Dietary fiber: 1.3 g, Sodium: 469 mg, Net carbs: 6.1 g, Carb Choice: ⅓

ANALYSIS FOR 1 SERVING:
½ cup made with Tofutti Better Than Sour Cream

Calories: 143, Fat: 8.4 g, Total carbohydrates: 11.2 g, Protein: 8.5 g,
Dietary fiber: 1.7 g, Sodium: 500 mg, Net carbs: 9.5 g, Carb Choice: ⅔

Three Sisters' Stew

MAKES 8½ CUPS; ABOUT 8 (1-CUP) SERVINGS

This hearty stew is a true Native American tradition. In the garden, the fabled "three sisters"— corn, beans, and squash—were planted together to help each other grow strong by giving nutrients and shade to one another. In a similar way, the three sisters provide sustenance and health protection to us humans, too. This stunning stew is richly flavored and nutritious as well.

1½ tablespoons Smart Balance Light Buttery Spread

1½ cups Morningstar Farms Grillers Recipe Crumbles, thawed, or other meatless burger crumbles

¾ cup chopped green bell pepper

1 cup chopped onion

2 cloves garlic, minced

3 cups water

1 (15-ounce) can regular-sodium canned pinto beans, drained (1½ cups)

1 (15-ounce) can regular-sodium, canned kidney beans, drained (1½ cups)

1 cup frozen whole-kernel yellow corn

2 cups ¾-inch cubes peeled butternut squash

2 tablespoons McKay's Beef-Style Instant Broth and Seasoning, Vegan

¾ teaspoon dried basil

¹/₁₆ teaspoon cayenne pepper

½ teaspoon salt

1 cup diced fresh tomato or low-sodium canned diced tomatoes

2 tablespoons water

1 tablespoon cornstarch

■ Melt the spread in a large pot over medium heat. Add the crumbles, pepper, onion, and garlic, and sauté until the vegetables are tender, 4 to 5 minutes. Add all the remaining ingredients, except the 2 tablespoons water and cornstarch. Cover and simmer until the vegetables are almost tender, about 20 minutes. Whisk the cornstarch and water together, and stir into the stew. Simmer for 5 minutes, stirring occasionally, and serve.

▶ *Nutrition Note:* This hearty stew has nutritional clout with its combination of beans, corn, and butternut squash. Once considered "poor man's food," beans are now known to be nutritional superstars. Besides their obvious versatility, they are rich in complex carbohydrates and low-fat protein (minus the harmful saturated fat and cholesterol found in meat). Beans are rich in soluble and insoluble fibers; the former helps to reduce the risk of heart disease by lowering LDL (bad) cholesterol levels. They also help to regulate blood sugar through their "low and slow" blood sugar rise. Beans are also a good source of the B vitamin thiamin, and an excellent source of the B vitamin folate. They are also mineral rich, including potassium, magnesium, selenium, and iron.

Yellow corn contains the two carotenoids lutein and xeaxanthin, both found in the macula of the human retina, and may help prevent age-related macular degeneration. Butternut squash is a gold mine of beta-carotene, the orange pigment that provides the body with vitamin A, as well as possessing antioxidant, immune-boosting, and cancer-fighting powers.

> **ANALYSIS FOR 1 SERVING:**
> 1 cup
>
> Calories: 163, Fat: 2.3 g, Total carbohydrates: 28.6 g, Protein: 9.1 g,
> Dietary fiber: 7.3 g, Sodium: 472 mg, Net carbs: 21.3 g, Carb Choice: 1⅓

Tofoo Yung

MAKES 11 PATTIES; ABOUT 5 (2-PATTY) SERVINGS

Our eggless, flourless, low-carb, high-fiber version of the Chinese favorite looks, smells, and tastes remarkably like the original thanks to the traditional vegetables and the versatility of tofu—and it isn't even fried!

1 tablespoon extra-virgin olive oil

½ cup fresh snow peas

½ cup fresh sliced mushrooms

½ cup thinly sliced onion

½ cup canned sliced bamboo shoots, drained

¾ cup canned sliced water chestnuts, drained

1 cup fresh bean sprouts

1 cup water-packed, extra-firm tofu, drained

1 tablespoon Bragg Liquid Aminos or low-sodium soy sauce

1½ tablespoons Red Star nutritional yeast flakes

2 teaspoons Ener-G Egg Replacer

¾ teaspoon salt

1 tablespoon Resource ThickenUp instant food thickener or other thickener

Asian Glaze (page 212) (optional)

■ Preheat the oven to 350°F. Spray a baking sheet with cooking spray. Heat the olive oil in a skillet over medium heat. Add the snow peas, mushrooms, onion, bamboo shoots, water chestnuts, and bean sprouts, and sauté until the onion is tender, 3 to 4 minutes.

■ Process the tofu and Bragg Liquid Aminos in a food processor until creamy, and transfer to a bowl. Stir in the sautéed vegetables and remaining ingredients and mix well. Measure ¼-cup portions, shape into patties, and place on prepared baking sheet. Bake for 15 minutes, turn, and bake for another 15 minutes, until firm and golden. Top each patty with 2 tablespoons Asian Glaze (if using).

ANALYSIS FOR 1 SERVING:
2 patties without glaze

Calories: 99, Fat: 5.1 g, Total carbohydrates: 8.5 g, Protein: 7.1 g,
Dietary fiber: 2.1 g, Sodium: 462 mg, Net carbs: 6.4 g, Carb Choice: ⅓

Tuscan Stuffed Peppers

MAKES 5 SERVINGS; 2 STUFFED PEPPER HALVES PER SERVING

Choose your favorite colored bell peppers and get stuffing! Our Tuscan peppers are filled with a medley of grilled fresh vegetables, with a sprinkling of toasted pine nuts on top. They're much lower-carb and lower-fat than traditional stuffed peppers, which are full of rice and ground meat.

5 large bell peppers (green, red, yellow, or a mixture)

1 tablespoon extra-virgin olive oil·

1 cup diced red onion

1 cup diced zucchini

1 cup diced yellow squash

½ cup sliced fresh mushrooms

1 cup diced fresh tomatoes

1 clove garlic, minced

⅓ cup pine nuts

¼ cup Chunky Marinara Sauce (page 216)

½ teaspoon salt

2 tablespoons dried basil

10 tablespoons Pimiento Cheese Sauce (page 228)

■ Preheat the oven to 350°F. Cut the peppers in half lengthwise and scoop out the seeds and ribs. Put cut-side down in baking dish filled with ¼-inch cold water. Place on a rack in a large pan and steam over boiling water for about 6 minutes. Remove the peppers with tongs and place on paper towels to drain.

■ Heat the olive oil in a skillet over medium heat. Add the vegetables and garlic and sauté for 3 to 4 minutes.

■ Meanwhile, toast the pine nuts by arranging them on an unsprayed baking sheet, and placing in the preheated oven for about 8 minutes, until browned and aromatic. Remove from the baking sheet and set aside. Fold the marinara sauce, pine nuts, salt, and basil into the vegetable mixture. Stuff each pepper half with ⅓ cup of the vegetable mixture. Top each pepper half with 1 tablespoon of the sauce. Bake for 30 minutes, stuffed side up, until the peppers are soft.

ANALYSIS FOR 1 SERVING:
2 stuffed pepper halves

Calories: 182, Fat: 9.9 g, Total carbohydrates: 21.3 g, Protein: 6.9 g, Dietary fiber: 5.0 g, Sodium: 440 mg, Net carbs: 16.3 g, Carb Choice: 1

Zesty Black Bean Soup

This is a spicy and bold soup, and because it is so hearty, one cup can serve as an entrée. Enjoy it with a slice of Ezekiel 4:9 Sprouted Grain bread, fresh green salad, and your favorite steamed veggie, and you'll be satisfied for hours.

1 tablespoon canola oil

1½ cups chopped onions

4 cloves garlic, chopped

1 teaspoon ground cumin

1 tablespoon chili powder

½ teaspoon dried oregano

⅛ teaspoon cayenne pepper

½ teaspoon salt

1 cup diced red bell pepper

½ cup diced yellow bell pepper

3 (15-ounce) cans low-sodium black beans, drained (4½ cups)

1½ cups water

5 teaspoons Tofu Sour Cream Supreme (page 235) or Tofutti Better Than Sour Cream (optional)

- Heat the oil in a large pot over medium heat. Add the onions and sauté until tender, 3 to 4 minutes. Stir in the garlic, cumin, chili powder, oregano, cayenne, salt, and diced peppers.
- Puree 1½ cups of the beans with half of the water in a blender on high, about 30 seconds. Add the bean mixture to the pot. Add the remaining water and remaining whole (unblended) beans to the pot and stir together. Reduce the heat and simmer for 15 minutes, stirring often. Garnish each serving with 1 teaspoon Tofu Sour Cream Supreme or Tofutti Better Than Sour Cream (if using).

ANALYSIS FOR 1 SERVING:
1 cup

Calories: 256, Fat: 3.9 g, Total carbohydrates: 44.5 g, Protein: 13.3 g,
Dietary fiber: 10.9 g, Sodium: 484 mg, Net carbs: 33.6 g, Carb Choice: 2

ANALYSIS FOR 1 SERVING:
1 cup with 1 teaspoon Tofu Sour Cream Supreme

Calories: 268, Fat: 4.7 g, Total carbohydrates: 45.4 g, Protein: 13.5 g,
Dietary fiber: 11.0 g, Sodium: 508 mg, Net carbs: 34.4 g, Carb Choice: 2

ANALYSIS FOR 1 SERVING:
1 cup with 1 teaspoon Tofutti Better Than Sour Cream

Calories: 272, Fat: 4.8 g, Total carbohydrates: 46.3 g, Protein: 13.5 g,
Dietary fiber: 11.1 g, Sodium: 514 mg, Net carbs: 35.2 g, Carb Choice: 2⅓

THERE'S AN OLD *Lockhorns* comic strip by Bunny Hoest and John Reiner (King Features Syndicate): Leroy looks up from his dinner plate and asks his wife, Loretta, "This side dish—whose side is it on?" For most side dishes on the Standard American Diet, that's a valid question. Typical side dishes like French fries, baked white potatoes with sour cream, white rice, and candied sweet potatoes tend to be mere extra bowls of fat, calories, sugar, and highly processed carbohydrates. They're hard to avoid: Studies show that the more side dishes and little bowls of extra goodies that are on the table, the more likely you will be to "graze" through them. Our side dishes, on the other hand, consist mainly of beans, whole grains, vegetables, and limited amounts of nuts. Their nutritional benefits necessitate our ennobling them, even elevating them to the level of traditional entrées. Our sides always *enhance* the nutritional value of an overall meal. They do so in several ways:

1. **They add fiber, especially those with beans, vegetables, and whole grains.** For example, ½ cup of cooked kidney beans, a fiber superfood, has 1.6 grams of soluble fiber and 4.9 grams of insoluble fiber. When it comes to vegetables, you get all the benefits of fiber (not the least of which is a feeling of satiety) from these miracle foods, which are naturally low in calories, fat, and sodium.

2. **They keep your blood sugar from spiking.** Those with beans, vegetables, and nuts add lower glycemic index (GI) choices to

balance the overall meal, thus ensuring your blood sugars don't rise as quickly or as high, even when some other choices in the meal might be higher glycemic.

3. **They add the right kind of protein.** Beans, nuts, and tofu are better sources of protein for you, and lower in calories than animal sources. While certain vegetables have protein, it's beans that are the "big daddy" of plant-based protein (26 percent of their calories come from protein—that's the same percentage as beef rib roast [fat trimmed to ⅛ inch]). To get the necessary full spectrum of essential proteins, simply eat a variety of plant-based foods, including a good selection of fruits, vegetables, whole grains, nuts, seeds, and beans.

4. **They add health-promoting vitamins, minerals, antioxidants, and phytochemicals.** These appear in nearly every whole grain, vegetable, legume (sprouts, beans, peas, soybeans), nut, and seed in a plant-based diet. They make you look good, they make you feel good, and they keep your body working properly.

5. **Those with legumes and vegetables help you lose weight, lower your cholesterol and triglycerides, and keep your blood sugar and blood pressure under control.** They also boost your energy level, even while lowering your risk of certain cancers, stroke, and heart disease, and helping to prevent, stop, and reverse diabetes.

FRESH VEGETABLE NOTES

- Every vegetable has its own unique mix of essential vitamins and minerals.
- A good variety of vegetables will cover all the nutrients you need.
- The fresher the better, so buy from local farmers markets, organic markets, or a trusted greengrocer.
- If moldy, throw the whole food away. Never cut a portion off and eat the rest.
- When possible, eat produce in season.
- Hand-pick your produce. Prepackaged bags of produce often contain inferior product. Squeeze, sniff, and inspect for freshness.
- Wash well. Scrub, don't soak. Use cold soapy water or an organic cleaner like Veggie Wash. Rinse well.
- Don't peel if you don't have to.
- Use fresh in season first, frozen second, and canned third.

CHOOSING FRESH VEGETABLES

Asparagus

Thickness is a matter of taste. Choose bunches with tightly closed, nonflowering tips. Stalks should be bright green and firm. Avoid those with stalks that are flattened, wrinkled, or hollow.

Avocados

Yes, they're fruits, but we've included them here because they're not sweet, and we don't use them as dessert foods. Look for avocados with bumpy, dark-green to almost-black skin. When ripe, they will give to gentle pressure (pressing too hard will bruise the flesh). If you buy firm, store it at room temperature to ripen, or if you're in a hurry, place in a sealed brown paper bag.

Corn

Best served the day you buy it. Don't refrigerate. Bright-green husks wrapped tightly around ear, with flowing, moist silk (not brown). Pull the husk back slighty: Kernels should be small, shiny, firm, and tightly packed. If a kernel sprays a little white liquid when pierced, it's just right.

Cucumbers

Look for firm, unwaxed varieties, with variegated color from light to dark green, and without wrinkles or soft spots.

Eggplant

Skin should be shiny, not shriveled, wrinkled, or mottled. Stems should be green. Use within a day or two. Don't refrigerate.

Green beans

Pole beans should be bright and firm with no soft spots or wrinkles. They should snap when bent. Avoid tough skin. Pods should be a bit leathery and firm, with no yellowing. Beans should be easily felt through the pod.

Lettuces and greens

There should be no wilted leaves, or wet, mushy, yellow spots. Romaine lettuce should have dark green, narrow, stiff leaves. Butter lettuces should have small, round, loosely formed heads.

Onions

Look for dry, papery skins and flesh that is full and firm, especially at the stem end. Avoid any with mold, discoloration, or soft spots. Store at room temperature.

Peppers

Bell peppers should be very firm all over with taut skin. Flesh should be thick without soft spots or wrinkles. Look for bright green stems. Chilies of all colors should be vibrant-looking and wrinkle-free.

Potatoes

All varieties should be firm, without any soft areas or wrinkled skin. Avoid those with sprouting eyes, slits, or a green tinge. Store at room temperature.

Squash

Yellow and green summer varieties should be small to medium, 5 to 6 inches and not bulbous (larger summer squashes are watery or fibrous). Should feel firm. Skin should be smooth and shiny.

Tomatoes

Yes, technically they're fruits, but we've included them here because we don't use them as dessert foods. Should be firm but not hard, with uniform, bright color, taut skin, and no blemishes. Best in season, from farm stands and farmers markets. Do not refrigerate. To ripen quickly, place in a brown paper bag.

COOKING FRESH VEGETABLES

IMPROPERLY COOKED VEGETABLES can lose their colors, flavors, and nutritional value. Following are some healthy ways to cook vegetables:

Steaming

Wash, trim, and cut into desired size. Arrange the vegetables in the cradle of the steamer and place in a covered pot with 1 inch of water in the bottom. You can save the liquid after steaming and use it for stock.

Baking or Roasting

Preheat oven to 350°F. Wash, trim, and cut into desired size. Place vegetables in a bowl and spray for 3 to 6 seconds with olive oil or another cooking spray. Sprinkle with your choice of seasonings, mix well, and place on a sprayed baking sheet in preheated oven. Bake until desired tenderness.

Grilling

Preheat grill to low-medium. Wash, trim, and cut into desired size. Soak in cold water or a low-fat marinade for 20 to 30 minutes (you can use diluted low-sodium soy sauce). Pat dry and brush lightly with seasoned oil. Make sure that your grill surface is clean, or use a grill basket if you don't want to place the food directly on the grill itself. Spray with your choice of vegetable cooking sprays to avoid sticking. Asparagus, corn, peppers, zucchini, onions, eggplant, tomatoes, mushrooms, and green beans are some of our favorites to grill. Turn often to grill all sides of the food. Remove when the desired doneness and look is achieved. Every vegetable will require a different time, depending on thickness.

DON'T GO NUTS

AGAIN, IT'S IMPORTANT to watch your side dish portions, of course. This is particularly true when it comes to nuts. As opposed to beans and vegetables, which are nearly fat-free, nuts have enough calories and fat, albeit mostly healthy unsaturated fat, to sabotage your health goals if you eat too many. For optimal health, eat nuts every day, but don't go nuts. We recommend eating no more than 1 ounce of nuts and/or seeds per day (or 2 tablespoons nut butter). If you need to lose weight, you should have no more than ½ ounce of nuts and/or seeds per day or 1 tablespoon nut butter.

NUTRIENTS IN 1 OUNCE OF RAW NUTS

Type of Nuts	Number of Nuts/Ounce	Calories	Fat (g)	Protein (g)	Carbo-hydrate (g)	Fiber (g)
Almonds	23 (scant ¼ cup)	164	14.4	6.0	5.6	3.3
Brazil nuts	6 to 8 (2 to 2½ tablespoons)	186	18.8	4.1	3.5	2.1
Cashews, whole	17 (¼ cup)	157	12.4	5.2	8.6	0.9
Hazelnuts	21 (scant ¼ cup)	178	17.2	4.2	4.7	2.7
Macadamias	10–12 (scant ¼ cup)	204	21.5	2.2	3.9	2.4
Peanuts (Valencia)	28 (2½ tablespoons)	162	14.1	7.2	4.5	2.7
Pecan halves	20 (¼ cup)	196	20.4	2.6	3.9	2.7
Pine nuts	15 to 16	160	14.4	6.8	4.0	1.3
Pistachios	47 (3½ tablespoons)	158	12.6	5.8	7.9	2.9
Walnut halves	14 (scant ½ cup)	185	18.5	4.3	3.9	1.9

NUTRIENTS IN 1 TABLESPOON NUT OR SEED BUTTERS

Type of Nut or Seed Butter	Amount	Calories	Fat (g)	Protein (g)	Carbo- hydrate (g)	Fiber (g)
Almond	1 tablespoon	101	9.5	2.4	3.4	0.6
Cashew	1 tablespoon	94	7.9	2.8	4.4	0.3
Macadamia	1 tablespoon	115	12.0	1.5	2.5	1.5
Peanut creamy/chunky	1 tablespoon	95	8.0	3.5	4.0	1.0
Sesame (Tahini)	1 tablespoon	89	8.1	2.6	3.2	1.4
Sunflower	1 tablespoon	93	7.6	3.1	4.4	—
Soy creamy/chunky	1 tablespoon	80	6.5	4.0	2.5	2.5

NUTRIENTS IN 1 OUNCE RAW SEEDS

Type of Seed	Amount for 1 ounce	Calories (Kcal)	Fat (g)	Protein (g)	Carbo- hydrate (g)	Fiber (g)
Flax	2 tablespoons	110	8.7	3.8	5.9	5.6
Pumpkin	2 tablespoons	153	13.9	7.0	5.1	1.1
Sesame	3 tablespoons plus ½ teaspoon	160	13.6	4.8	7.3	4.0
Sunflower	¼ cup	165	14.1	5.5	6.8	2.6

Source: USDA National Nutrient Database for Standard Reference, Release 18, available at www.ars.usda.gov/ba/bhnrc/ndl and www.nal.usda.gov/fnic/foodcomp.

Abuela Amelia's Beans

MAKES 6²⁄₃ CUPS; ABOUT 13 (½-CUP) SERVINGS

This recipe, an LCA favorite, comes from our resident "grandma," Amelia, who assists Linda K. in our cooking school. The humble, mottled pinto bean, a staple of the Southwestern and Mexican-American diet, is the basis of this high-fiber side dish. If you don't have a pressure cooker, you can make this recipe starting with 6 cups cooked pinto beans that have been pre-cooked by another method—slow cooker, stovetop, or even canned. See table on page 10 for additional directions.

2 cups dry pinto beans, soaked overnight (see page 59)

3 cups water

½ teaspoon salt

1 tablespoon extra-virgin olive oil

1 cup chopped onion

¼ cup chopped green bell pepper

3 cloves garlic, minced

¾ cup chopped tomatoes

2 tablespoons tomato paste

1 tablespoon McKay's Beef-Style Instant Broth and Seasoning, Vegan

½ teaspoon dried oregano

½ teaspoon dried basil

¼ teaspoon ground cumin

1 bay leaf

½ teaspoon salt

■ Cook the beans, water, and salt in a pressure cooker according to manufacturer's directions until the beans are tender. You will end up with 6 cups of cooked beans.

■ Heat the olive oil in a small skillet over medium heat. Add the onion, pepper, and garlic, and sauté until onion is tender, 4 to 5 minutes. Add to the beans. Stir in the remaining ingredients, and simmer for 15 minutes. You may smash some of the cooked beans against the side of the pot to make the beans saucy. Leftover beans can be refrigerated for up to 3 days or frozen for up to 1 month.

ANALYSIS FOR 1 SERVING:
½ cup

Calories: 127, Fat: 1.5 g, Total carbohydrates: 22.6 g, Protein: 6.8 g,
Dietary fiber: 7.2 g, Sodium: 243 mg, Net carbs: 15.4 g, Carb Choice: 1

Baked Sweet Potato

Sweet potatoes are a very nutritious substitute for white potatoes, with nearly 20 percent fewer carbs, 40 percent fewer calories, and close to twice the fiber of russet potatoes. But in fact, sweet potatoes aren't even related to potatoes. They're also not related to yams, though in the American South, the terms are interchangeable.

1 medium sweet potato (7–8 ounces)   Cooking spray

■ Preheat oven to 350°F. Spray a baking sheet with cooking spray. Peel the sweet potato, cut into 4 pieces, and place on prepared baking sheet. Spray the potato pieces with cooking spray for 1 second. Bake for 30 to 35 minutes, until tender.

▶ *Nutrition Note:* Sweet potatoes are edible roots, not tubers like white potatoes. They're members of the morning glory family, while white potatoes are actually nightshades. Sweet potatoes are lower glycemic than white potatoes. See Nutrition Note for Sweet Potato Fries (page 203) to learn more about sweet potatoes.

ANALYSIS FOR 1 SERVING:
½ of the potato (2 pieces) with cooking spray

Calories: 65, Fat: 0.8 g, Total carbohydrates: 13.8 g, Protein: 1.0 g,
Dietary fiber: 1.7 g, Sodium: 6 mg, Net carbs: 12.1 g, Carb Choice: ⅔

Brilliant Kale with Red Pepper and Onion

Kale is a high-protein, phytochemical king, with a more intense flavor than most other vegetables. Because kale can taste bitter when cooked improperly, we recommend this double-cooking method of boiling, then sautéing, which pacifies the sharpness of this green. The result is a mild, semisweet, cabbagelike flavor, divine when embellished with sweet red bell pepper and onion. Wash kale well, but don't soak. If leaves are small, do not chop. If leaves are larger, remove the coarsest part of the stem, and stack 6 to 8 leaves on top of one another. Cut crosswise into 1-inch strips.

5 cups water

8 cups coarsely chopped fresh kale

½ teaspoon extra-virgin olive oil

½ cup thinly sliced onion

¼ cup red bell pepper strips

1 teaspoon minced garlic

1 teaspoon McKay's Chicken-Style Instant Broth and Seasoning, Vegan

½ tablespoon Red Star nutritional yeast flakes

■ In a large pot, bring the water to a boil, add the kale, and cook briefly until it turns bright green. Drain and set aside. Heat the oil in a saucepan over medium heat, add the onion, bell pepper, and garlic, and sauté until tender, 4 to 5 minutes. Add the kale and increase the heat to medium-high, toss with vegetables, and sauté for 4 to 5 minutes. Add the seasonings and yeast, stir well, and serve.

▶ *Nutrition Note:* It s time to take kale out of its "garnish" status and put it in the superfood category. Kale gives broccoli a run for its money, with 7 times more beta-carotene than broccoli, and almost 11 times more lutein, a carotenoid found in the macula of the human retina and believed to reduce the risk of age-related macular degeneration, a major cause of visual impairment in the United States. Kale also contains respectable amounts of xeaxanthin, another carotenoid that may combat macular degeneration.

> **ANALYSIS FOR 1 SERVING:**
> 1 cup
>
> Calories: 127, Fat: 2.7 g, Total carbohydrates: 21.2 g, Protein: 10.3 g, Dietary fiber: 7.2 g, Sodium: 65 mg, Net carbs: 14 g, Carb Choice: 1

Cauliflower Mashed Potatoes

*S*top the presses—we have great news for people with diabetes! This recipe looks, smells, and tastes like authentic mashed potatoes, but it's much lower glycemic than the traditional dish, so often relegated to the "do not eat" list for people with diabetes. The secret is a 2:1 ratio of mashed cauliflower to mashed potato. It's a surprisingly happy union that doesn't even need gravy. Serve with our Savory Dinner Roast (page 157) or any dish begging for the unmistakably creamy addition of mashed potatoes. And if you just can't forgo the gravy, try these with our Windcrest Country Gravy (page 237). Do not use soymilk that has been sweetened. Even "plain" soymilk is often sweetened, so read the label carefully as sweetened soymilk alters the flavor of this recipe significantly. Also note that when you overprocess or overblend potatoes, their starches break down even more, causing a "gluey" consistency.

2 cups coarsely chopped fresh cauliflower florets

1 cup 1-inch peeled red potato cubes

2 tablespoons unsweetened soymilk

1 tablespoon Smart Balance Light Buttery Spread

½ teaspoon garlic powder

¼ teaspoon salt, or to taste

■ In a steamer basket set over boiling water, steam the cauliflower and potatoes together until soft, about 12 minutes. Place the hot vegetables and all remaining ingredients into a food processor, and puree on high for 15 to 30 seconds, or until smooth. Stop the processor before the potatoes become "gluey."

ANALYSIS FOR 1 SERVING:
¾ cup

Calories: 89, Fat: 2.3 g, Total carbohydrates: 15.6 g, Protein: 2.9 g,
Dietary fiber: 3.0 g, Sodium: 282 mg, Net carbs: 12.6 g, Carb Choice: 1

Cinnamon Yam Smash

Is a yam the same thing as a sweet potato? When Southern folks encounter Yankees at Windcrest Restaurant, they take this subject so seriously you'd think it would come to fisticuffs. No matter though; with a tinge of cinnamon and maple syrup, this recipe shines whether you call them sweet potatoes or yams.

5 medium sweet potatoes (7–8 ounces each)

1 teaspoon frozen white grape juice concentrate

2 teaspoons maple syrup or ½–1 teaspoon maple flavoring

1 teaspoon ground cinnamon

2 tablespoons Smart Balance Light Buttery Spread

■ Preheat the oven to 400°F. Bake the sweet potatoes for 50 minutes, until soft to the touch. Cool enough to handle, peel, and place in a large, flat-bottom dish. Add all remaining ingredients and mash until desired consistency. Serve hot.

▶ *Nutrition Note:* While the amount of maple syrup in this recipe is negligible, you may choose to leave it out and use the maple flavoring: you will get the coloring and flavor you need, without the carbs. Also, while the words *sweet potato* and *yam* are often used interchangeably, they belong to two different botanical families: sweet potatoes from the morning glory family, yams from the lily family. Yams are large root vegetables grown mainly in Africa, South America, or the Caribbean, with more than 600 different species. Yams tend to be slightly less flavorful, and drier than sweet potatoes, and contain less beta-carotene.

ANALYSIS FOR 1 SERVING:
½ cup made with maple syrup

Calories: 120, Fat: 1.8 g, Total carbohydrates: 25 g, Protein: 1.7 g, Dietary fiber: 3.1 g, Sodium: 38 mg, Net carbs: 21.9 g, Carb Choice: 1½

ANALYSIS FOR 1 SERVING:
½ cup made with maple flavoring

Calories: 116, Fat: 1.8 g, Total carbohydrates: 23.6 g, Protein: 1.7 g, Dietary fiber: 3.1 g, Sodium: 38 mg, Net carbs: 20.5 g, Carb Choice: 1⅓

Southern Country Cornbread

MAKES 16 (2-INCH) SQUARES

There's no more Southern meal than a bowl of savory chili beans accompanied by a piece of hearty warm cornbread. We use no dairy and whole grain cornmeal, which makes a substantial cornbread, even while ensuring it's lower glycemic and healthier than traditional cornbread made with highly processed cornmeal, white flour, eggs, butter, sour cream, or buttermilk. Extra pieces freeze well. Because whole grains tend to be heavier than refined (processed) grains, using whole grain cornmeal works well in this recipe. Southern cornbread's supposed to be dense, not light and fluffy. However, we don't suggest using coarse-grind cornmeal, as this would produce too dense and gritty a cornbread.

1 cup Bob's Red Mill whole grain cornmeal or other whole grain cornmeal, fine or medium grind

1¼ cups whole wheat pastry flour or barley flour

½ teaspoon salt

1 tablespoon Rumford baking powder

2 tablespoons 100 percent natural floral honey

2 tablespoons canola oil

¾ cup water

½ cup Silk unsweetened or plain soymilk

¼ cup Mori-Nu lite, firm silken tofu

2 teaspoons vanilla extract (optional)

■ Preheat the oven to 350°F. Spray an 8-inch-square baking dish with cooking spray. In a bowl, stir together the cornmeal, flour, salt, and baking powder. In a blender on medium, blend the honey, canola oil, water, soymilk, tofu, and vanilla until creamy, about 45 seconds. Add wet ingredients to the dry and stir together quickly. Spoon into prepared baking dish, gently shake pan to level the batter, and immediately place in the oven. For a moister cornbread, place a pan of water on the rack underneath the baking pan. Bake for 40 to 45 minutes. Cool and cut into squares.

ANALYSIS FOR 1 SERVING:
1 (2-inch) square

Calories: 95, Fat: 2.3 g, Total carbohydrates: 16.7 g, Protein: 2.6 g,
Dietary fiber: 2.0 g, Sodium: 241 mg, Net carbs: 14.9 g, Carb Choice: 1

Confetti Cornbread

MAKES 16 (2-INCH) SQUARES

This is a Tex-Mex variation of our Southern Country Cornbread (opposite), with an added splash of color. Extra pieces freeze well. Though Southern-style cornbread is supposed to be dense, not fluffy, we don't suggest using coarse-grind cornmeal, as this would produce too dense and gritty a cornbread.

1 cup Bob's Red Mill whole grain cornmeal or other whole grain cornmeal, fine or medium grind

1¼ cups whole wheat pastry flour

½ teaspoon salt

1 tablespoon Rumford baking powder

1 teaspoon chili powder

¼ teaspoon ground cumin

2 tablespoons 100 percent natural floral honey

2 tablespoons canola oil

¾ cup water

½ cup Silk unsweetened or plain soymilk

¼ cup Mori-Nu lite, firm silken tofu

1 (4.5-ounce) can diced mild green chilies, drained

1 (2-ounce) jar diced pimientos, drained (¼ cup)

1 whole jalapeño chili, seeds removed, and finely chopped

¼ cup frozen whole-kernel yellow corn

■ Preheat the oven to 350°F. Spray an 8-inch-square baking dish with cooking spray. In a bowl, stir together the cornmeal, flour, salt, baking powder, chili powder, and cumin. In a blender on medium, blend the honey, oil, water, soymilk, and tofu until creamy, about 45 seconds. Pour wet mixture into a bowl. Add the green chilies, pimientos, jalapeño chili, and corn, and stir together. Combine the wet and dry ingredients quickly and pour into prepared baking dish. Gently shake pan to level the batter and immediately put in the oven. For a moister cornbread, place a pan of water on the rack underneath the baking pan. Bake for 40 to 45 minutes. Cool and cut into squares.

ANALYSIS FOR 1 SERVING:
1 (2-inch) square

Calories: 96, Fat: 2.4 g, Total carbohydrates: 17.4 g, Protein: 2.7 g, Dietary fiber: 2.4 g, Sodium: 273 mg, Net carbs: 15 g, Carb Choice: 1

Curried Garbanzos

Coconut milk, curry, and cumin gives this popular Indian dish a rich, spicy flavor, but you'll find this version much milder than most traditional curry dishes.

1 tablespoon canola oil

1 teaspoon cumin seed

1½ cups finely chopped onions

2 cloves garlic, minced

1 (14.5-ounce) can crushed tomatoes

2 (15-ounce) cans regular-sodium garbanzo beans, drained (3 cups)

½ jalapeño chili, seeds removed, and finely diced

1 teaspoon curry powder

1 teaspoon salt

½ cup reduced-fat coconut milk

¼ cup chopped fresh cilantro

■ Heat the oil in a large skillet over medium heat. Add the cumin seed and cook until they begin to pop, about 30 seconds. Quickly add the onions and cook until they begin to brown, 3 to 4 minutes. Add the garlic and cook for 1 minute. Add the tomatoes, beans, jalapeño chili, curry powder, salt, and coconut milk. Reduce the heat to low and simmer for 10 minutes. Stir in the cilantro just before serving.

ANALYSIS FOR 1 SERVING:
½ cup

Calories: 151, Fat: 4.5 g, Total carbohydrates: 22.7 g, Protein: 6.6 g,
Dietary fiber: 6.0 g, Sodium: 309 mg, Net carbs: 16.7 g, Carb Choice: 1

Garbanzo Medley

This recipe unites garbanzos together with summer and winter squashes for a satisfying dish that's bursting with color and flavor, but not with carbs, calories, or fat. This medley may be used as a side, or served with a leafy green salad as a meal.

1 cup ½-inch carrot pieces

2 cups ½-inch zucchini pieces

½ cup ½-inch peeled butternut squash pieces

¾ teaspoon extra-virgin olive oil

½ cup thinly sliced onion

1 clove garlic, minced

½ teaspoon ground coriander

½ teaspoon McKay's Chicken-Style Instant Broth and Seasoning, Vegan

¼ teaspoon salt

⅛ teaspoon sweet paprika

1 cup regular-sodium canned garbanzo beans, drained

■ Steam the carrot, zucchini, and butternut squash until almost done, 10 to 12 minutes. Heat the oil in a medium saucepan over medium heat. Add the onion and garlic and sauté until tender, 3 to 4 minutes. Add the steamed vegetables and remaining ingredients, and cook until the vegetables are done, 8 to 10 minutes more. Serve hot.

ANALYSIS FOR 1 SERVING:
½ cup

Calories: 56, Fat: 1.1 g, Total carbohydrates: 9.8 g, Protein: 2.5 g, Dietary fiber: 2.8 g, Sodium: 111 mg, Net carbs: 7 g, Carb Choice: ½

Seasoned Garbanzos

The unassuming but nutrient-dense garbanzo bean is the basis for this appetizing side dish, one of the most popular bean dishes we make at LCA. Its weighty taste, muscular texture, and high-protein content remind our guests you don't need meat to make a meal.

¾ teaspoon canola oil

¼ cup diced onion

¼ cup diced carrot

2 (15-ounce) cans regular-sodium garbanzo beans, drained (3 cups)

1 cup water

1 tablespoon Red Star nutritional yeast flakes

⅛ teaspoon turmeric powder

½ teaspoon seasoned salt

¼ teaspoon garlic powder

¼ teaspoon onion powder

½ teaspoon low-sodium soy sauce

⅛ teaspoon curry powder

■ Heat the oil in a medium pot over medium heat. Add the onion and carrot and sauté until tender, 3 to 4 minutes. Add the remaining ingredients and simmer until the carrot is tender, 15 to 20 minutes. Serve hot. Leftover beans can be refrigerated for up to 3 days or frozen for up to 1 month.

ANALYSIS FOR 1 SERVING:
½ cup

Calories: 151, Fat: 2.7 g, Total carbohydrates: 24.5 g, Protein: 8.4 g, Dietary fiber: 6.9 g, Sodium: 244 mg, Net carbs: 17.6 g, Carb Choice: 1

Great Northern Beans

Great Northern beans are white, mild-flavored, thin-skinned, and light. They're popular in Mediterranean cooking, in French cassoulet, and in America, baked and in soups. Here we bathe them in a seasoned broth for a protein- and fiber-filled side dish that lives up to this bean's name. You can substitute cannellini beans if Great Northerns are not available.

1 teaspoon extra-virgin olive oil

2 cups diced onions

5½ cups regular-sodium canned Great Northern beans, drained

2 cups water

1 bay leaf

1 teaspoon onion powder

½ teaspoon garlic powder

1½ teaspoons low-sodium soy sauce

½ teaspoon salt

1 tablespoon Red Star nutritional yeast flakes

1½ teaspoons McKay's Chicken-Style Instant Broth and Seasoning, Vegan

⅛ teaspoon dried thyme

■ Heat the oil in a medium saucepan over medium heat. Add the onions and sauté until tender, 3 to 4 minutes. Stir in the remaining ingredients and heat through. Leftover beans can be refrigerated for up to 3 days or frozen for up to 1 month.

ANALYSIS FOR 1 SERVING:
½ cup

Calories: 138, Fat: 1.5 g, Total carbohydrates: 23.6 g, Protein: 8.8 g, Dietary fiber: 5.8 g, Sodium: 129 mg, Net carbs: 17.8 g, Carb Choice: 1

Lima Beans

Called butter beans in the South and limas in the North (and "Madagascar beans" in other parts of the world), these beans are actually native to Peru, from whose capital city they derive their name. Lima beans have a mild, buttery flavor, hence their nickname. Here the juxtaposition of sharp pimiento and humble lima flavors puts a twist on an old standby. If you haven't tried lima beans since shunning them in childhood, give them a fair shake now that your tastes have matured. You can purchase lima beans in two sizes, "large, or Fordhook" and "baby." While devotees swear by one or the other, they can be interchanged in most recipes.

4 cups frozen baby lima beans

2 cups water

1 tablespoon Red Star nutritional yeast flakes

2 teaspoons McKay's Chicken-Style Instant Broth and Seasoning, Vegan

1½ teaspoons extra-virgin olive oil

6 tablespoons chopped onion

2 tablespoons canned diced pimientos, drained

■ Boil the limas, water, nutritional yeast, and chicken-style seasoning in a large saucepan until the beans are tender, 15 to 20 minutes. Heat the olive oil in a small skillet over medium heat. Add the onion and pimientos and sauté until the onion is tender, 3 to 4 minutes. Add to the beans and simmer until the sauce is creamy, about 10 minutes. As you stir, some beans will break apart to form a creamy sauce. Serve hot. Leftover beans can be refrigerated for up to 3 days or frozen for up to 1 month.

ANALYSIS FOR 1 SERVING:
½ cup

Calories: 116, Fat: 1.4 g, Total carbohydrates: 20.2 g, Protein: 6.8 g, Dietary fiber: 6.1 g, Sodium: 61 mg, Net carbs: 14.1 g, Carb Choice: 1

Edamame

These fabulous bright green soybeans are a staple of the Japanese diet. Our version calls for the high-protein gems to be cooked in a savory broth. Edamame can be eaten as an appetizer, side dish, or entrée.

½ teaspoon extra-virgin olive oil

¾ cup chopped onion

1 clove garlic, minced

4¼ cups frozen shelled edamame

2½ cups water

2½ tablespoons Red Star nutritional yeast flakes

1 tablespoon McKay's Chicken-Style Instant Broth and Seasoning, Vegan

½ teaspoon garlic powder

½ teaspoon onion powder

■ Heat the olive oil in a saucepan over medium heat. Add the onion and garlic and sauté until the onion is tender, 3 to 4 minutes. Add the remaining ingredients and simmer, covered, until the beans are tender, about 40 minutes.

ANALYSIS FOR 1 SERVING:
½ cup

Calories: 173 g, Fat: 7.2 g, Total carbohydrates: 15.5 g, Protein: 15.2 g, Dietary fiber: 5.5 g, Sodium: 28 mg, Net carbs: 10 g, Carb Choice: ⅔

Saucy Red Kidney Beans

*K*idney beans are a beautiful burgundy red and, unlike other beans, hold their shape well when cooked. They are legion in salads, Mexican dishes, and Tex-Mex dishes, and here they're simply seasoned and served as a satisfying side dish.

2 teaspoons extra-virgin olive oil

⅓ cup chopped onion

⅓ cup chopped green bell pepper

3⅓ cups regular-sodium canned kidney beans, drained

1 cup water

⅔ cup diced fresh tomatoes

⅛ teaspoon dried oregano leaves

½ teaspoon dried basil

⅛ teaspoon salt

¼ teaspoon garlic powder

■ Heat the oil in a medium saucepan over medium heat. Add the onion and pepper and sauté until tender, 4 to 5 minutes. Add the remaining ingredients and simmer for 10 minutes. Serve hot. Leftover beans can be refrigerated for up to 3 days or frozen for up to 1 month.

ANALYSIS FOR 1 SERVING:
½ cup

Calories: 99, Fat: 1.4 g, Total carbohydrates: 16.5 g, Protein: 5.9 g,
Dietary fiber: 4.6 g, Sodium: 191 mg, Net carbs: 12.1 g, Carb Choice: 1

Refried Frijoles Negros

Here's a quick and easy way to create refried beans with faithful Mexican flavor—and low-fat content (traditional refried beans are made with lard). Toasting the dry oregano leaves releases the flavorful oils, which then permeate these beans. Enjoy on our Pita Pizza with Refried Frijoles Negros (page 155) or Grilled Quesadilla (page 139). Pinto beans also work well in this recipe.

1 (15-ounce) can low-sodium black beans, drained (1½ cups)
½ cup water
1 teaspoon dried oregano leaves
1 tablespoon dried minced onion

½ teaspoon garlic powder
½ teaspoon extra-virgin olive oil
1/16 teaspoon cayenne pepper
1 teaspoon ground cumin

- Place the beans and water in a medium skillet over medium heat. In a small dry skillet over medium-high heat, toast the dried oregano for about 2 minutes, stirring constantly. Add the oregano and the remaining ingredients to the beans. Bring to a boil and mash with a potato masher until smooth. Leftover beans can be refrigerated for up to 3 days or frozen for up to 1 month.

ANALYSIS FOR 1 SERVING:
2 tablespoons

Calories: 42, Fat: 0.8 g, Total carbohydrates: 6.7 g, Protein: 2.2 g,
Dietary fiber: 1.6 g, Sodium: 56 mg, Net carbs: 5.1 g, Carb Choice: ⅓

Refried Pinto Beans

MAKES 4 CUPS; 8 (½-CUP) SERVINGS

This hardy little drought-resistant bean is the standard-bearer bean of the American Southwest, Mexico, and most Spanish-speaking countries, where it's the usual suspect in chili and refried beans. This low-fat, big-flavor refried pinto bean recipe is the basis for a lot of admired meals at Windcrest Restaurant. Eat as a side dish with Mexican food, or spread on an Ezekiel 4:9 tortilla or other whole wheat tortilla.

1½ teaspoons extra-virgin olive oil

¾ cup chopped onion

2 cloves garlic, minced

1½ teaspoons chili powder

1 teaspoon McKay's Beef-Style Instant Broth and Seasoning, Vegan

¼ teaspoon salt

⅛ teaspoon cayenne pepper

½ cup chopped fresh tomato

4 cups regular-sodium canned pinto beans, drained

■ Heat the oil in a medium skillet over medium heat. Add the onion and garlic and sauté until tender, 3 to 4 minutes. Add the seasonings and tomato, and cook for 2 to 3 minutes. Place the beans in a food processor, add the contents of the skillet, and process on medium setting until smooth. Return the bean mixture to the skillet and simmer on medium heat until the beans are thickened, about 10 minutes. Serve hot. Leftover beans can be refrigerated for up to 3 days or frozen for up to 1 month.

ANALYSIS FOR 1 SERVING:
½ cup

Calories: 135, Fat: 1.4 g, Total carbohydrates: 24.2 g, Protein: 7.4 g,
Dietary fiber: 7.9 g, Sodium: 241 mg, Net carbs: 16.3 g, Carb Choice: 1

Smoky Lentils with Caramelized Onions

Lentils have been indispensable fare in the Middle East, the Mediterranean, and India for millennia. But there's hardly a land in the world without its own favorite lentil-based specialty. Topped with caramelized onions, ours has a hint of smoked flavoring.

2 cups dry brown lentils	½ teaspoon liquid smoke
1 cup chopped onion	½ teaspoon salt
4 cups water	1½ teaspoons canola oil
1 tablespoon McKay's Beef-Style Instant Broth and Seasoning, Vegan	2 cups thinly sliced onion rings

- In a medium saucepan, bring the lentils, chopped onion, and water to a boil. Add seasonings, reduce the heat, cover, and simmer until tender, about 30 minutes.
- While the lentils are cooking, heat the oil in a skillet over medium heat. Add the sliced onions and sauté, stirring occasionally, about 8 minutes. Onions will turn dark brown with a syrupy juice. Top cooked lentils with caramelized onions and serve. Leftover lentils can be refrigerated for up to 3 days or frozen for up to 1 month.

ANALYSIS FOR 1 SERVING:
½ cup

Calories: 130, Fat: 1.0 g, Total carbohydrates: 22.8 g, Protein: 8.7 g, Dietary fiber: 7.7 g, Sodium: 149 mg, Net carbs: 15.1, Carb Choice: 1

Tasty Black-Eyed Peas

MAKES 4 CUPS; 8 (½-CUP) SERVINGS

Also known as "black-eyed beans" or "cowpeas," these beauties have become synonymous with "down-home" Southern cooking, though they're thought to have arrived from Asia via the African slave trade (they're still popular in Chinese cooking). This low-fat dish is mildly sweet, and begs to be eaten with a piece of our Southern Country Cornbread (page 180) or Confetti Cornbread (page 181).

½ teaspoon extra-virgin olive oil

½ cup chopped onion

¼ cup chopped celery

1 clove garlic, minced

3½ cups regular-sodium canned black-eyed peas, drained

1½ cups water

1½ teaspoons light molasses

¼ teaspoon dried oregano leaves

1½ teaspoons McKay's Chicken-Style Instant Broth and Seasoning, Vegan

¾ teaspoon seasoned salt

1 tablespoon canned tomato paste

■ Heat the oil in a medium saucepan over medium heat. Add the onion, celery, and garlic and sauté until tender, 4 to 5 minutes. Stir in the remaining ingredients. Simmer for 15 minutes to blend flavors. Smash about one-third of the peas against the side of the pot to make the dish saucy. Serve hot. Leftover black-eyed peas can be refrigerated for up to 3 days or frozen for up to 1 month.

> **ANALYSIS FOR 1 SERVING:**
> ½ cup
>
> Calories: 101, Fat: 0.7 g, Total carbohydrates: 18.4 g, Protein: 6.1 g, Dietary fiber: 5.2 g, Sodium: 308 mg, Net carbs: 13.2 g, Carb Choice: 1

Ebony Wild Rice

*W*ild rice works wonderfully in a diabetic diet because it's low glycemic. Wild rice's dramatically long, black, slender grains have a distinctive nutty flavor and chewy texture that's uniquely North American. This nutritious dish will fill out many entrées, such as our Lemon-Basil Kabobs (page 144) or Mazidra (page 147).

2 cups water
¼ teaspoon salt

⅔ cup wild rice
1 clove garlic, minced

In a medium saucepan with a tight-fitting lid, bring all the ingredients to a boil and stir briefly. Cover, reduce the heat, and simmer until the water is absorbed, 40 to 45 minutes.

> *Nutrition Note:* Wild rice is not a true rice, but the seed of an aquatic grass from an entirely different botanical family. It contains more protein than other rice, and is a good source of several B vitamins, including niacin and B_6.

ANALYSIS FOR 1 SERVING:
⅓ cup

Calories: 72, Fat: 0.2 g, Total carbohydrates: 15.2 g, Protein: 2.9 g,
Dietary fiber: 1.3 g, Sodium: 101 mg, Net carbs: 13.9 g, Carb Choice: 1

Mellow Brown Rice

It's very simple: Brown rice is nutritionally better for you than white rice. For one thing, it's closer to the whole grain original, therefore it's higher in fiber and has a lower glycemic index than white rice. Our specially seasoned brown rice will guarantee you won't go back to plain white rice again. Freeze leftover rice in serving sizes for up to one month. To make brown rice properly, add 1 cup brown rice to 2 cups water in a medium saucepan, and bring to a boil. Cover and reduce the heat, and simmer for about 45 minutes or until the water is absorbed. Don't stir, or the rice will be gummy. If using Uncle Ben's converted brown rice, cooking time will be about 30 minutes.

1½ teaspoons extra-virgin olive oil

¼ cup diced onion

1 clove garlic, minced

2 cups cooked brown rice (no salt added)

⅛ teaspoon salt

¼ teaspoon McKay's Chicken-Style Instant Broth and Seasoning, Vegan

■ Heat the oil in a large skillet over medium heat. Add the onion and garlic and sauté until tender, 3 to 4 minutes. Stir in the rice and seasonings. Mix well. Heat through and serve hot.

▶ *Nutrition Note:* Brown rice still contains nutrient-dense layers of the whole rice grain, whereas the super-processing of white rice robs it of many essential nutrients.

ANALYSIS FOR 1 SERVING:
⅓ cup

Calories: 85, Fat: 1.7 g, Total carbohydrates: 15.7 g, Protein: 1.8 g,
Dietary fiber: 1.3 g, Sodium: 54 mg, Net carbs: 14.4 g, Carb Choice: 1

Two-Color Rice Combo

MAKES 3 CUPS; 9 (⅓-CUP) SERVINGS

Basmati's a fragrant, long-grain rice with Himalayan origins, popular in Indian cuisine. Here it's coupled with North American wild rice for a side dish that has a lower glycemic index than standard white rice, and is much more flavorful. Freeze leftover rice for those days when there's no time to cook. Do not use Uncle Ben's converted brown rice in this recipe, because it will cook too quickly and turn gummy.

2 cups water
¼ teaspoon salt

½ cup wild rice
½ cup brown basmati rice or other brown rice

- In a small saucepan, bring the water and salt to a boil. Stir in both kinds of rice and return to a boil. Reduce the heat, cover, and simmer until the water is absorbed and the rice is fluffy, 35 to 40 minutes. Do not stir while cooking or rice will get gummy. Remove from heat and serve hot.

ANALYSIS FOR 1 SERVING:
⅓ cup

Calories: 74, Fat: 0.4 g, Total carbohydrates: 15.4 g, Protein: 2.3 g,
Dietary fiber: 1.3 g, Sodium: 69 mg, Net carbs: 14.1 g, Carb Choice: 1

Polenta Squares

*P*olenta *is a traditional Italian cornmeal porridge, sometimes served soft, and sometimes allowed to set overnight, as it is here. A lower glycemic alternative to pasta, our whole grain polenta boasts a heavy-duty flavor, with a crispy outside and yielding inside. Complement it with savory toppings such as our Succulent Ratatouille (page 160) or the beans of your choice.*

3 cups water   1 cup whole grain cornmeal
½ teaspoon salt

■ Spray an 8-inch-square pan with cooking spray. Bring 2 cups of the water and the salt to a boil in a medium saucepan. In a small bowl, whisk together the remaining 1 cup water with the cornmeal, and stir into the boiling water. Reduce the heat to medium-low, cover, and simmer for 30 minutes, stirring occasionally. Pour the polenta into prepared dish, cover, and refrigerate overnight. Cut into 8 pieces.

■ Spray a large skillet with cooking spray and heat over medium-low heat. Add the polenta pieces and cook for 15 minutes on each side. Serve hot as a side dish or with toppings.

ANALYSIS FOR 1 SERVING:
⅛ of an 8-inch-square baking dish

Calories: 60, Fat: 0.6 g, Total carbohydrates: 12.6 g, Protein: 1.5 g,
Dietary fiber: 1.6 g, Sodium: 149 mg, Net carbs: 11 g, Carb Choice: ⅔

Rustic Quinoa Pilaf

*T*his low glycemic seed has a delightfully mild nutty flavor, with a light and fluffy consistency. The combination of herbs and spices makes this pilaf an excellent side dish to many entrées. Or you might find a steaming bowl is quite enough on its own. Leftovers freeze well. Rinse quinoa in a fine-mesh colander until the water becomes clear, in order to remove the bitter-tasting resin (saponin) on the quinoa.

1½ teaspoons extra-virgin olive oil

¾ cup frozen whole-kernel yellow corn

¼ cup finely diced red bell pepper

1 cup finely chopped onion

3 cloves garlic, minced

1 medium jalapeño chili, seeds removed, minced

1 cup quinoa, rinsed

½ teaspoon salt

2 cups hot water

2 teaspoons McKay's Chicken-Style Instant Broth and Seasoning, Vegan

¼ teaspoon celery salt

1 teaspoon grated lime zest

2 tablespoons chopped fresh cilantro

¾ teaspoon fresh lime juice

¹⁄₁₆ teaspoon cayenne pepper, or to taste

- Heat ½ teaspoon of the oil in a small skillet over medium heat. Add the corn and sauté, stirring frequently, until the corn browns, 2 to 3 minutes. Remove from heat and set aside.

- Heat the remaining 1 teaspoon oil in a large skillet over medium heat. Add the pepper, onion, garlic, and jalapeño chili and sauté until tender, 4 to 5 minutes. Add the quinoa and salt, and sauté on medium-high, stirring often, until the quinoa starts to brown, 5 to 8 minutes.

- In a small bowl, mix the hot water, chicken-style seasoning, celery salt, and lime zest. Add to the quinoa, bring to a boil, reduce the heat to low, and cook uncovered about 10 minutes. Cover and cook for 15 minutes. Remove from heat, place the lid ajar, and let stand for 10 minutes. Remove the lid, and fluff with a fork. Stir in the corn, cilantro, lime juice, and cayenne. Serve hot or cold. Leftover pilaf can be refrigerated for up to 3 days or frozen for up to 1 month.

▶ *Nutrition Note:* Quinoa's nutritional hallmark is its high level of lysine, an essential amino acid necessary for protein synthesis. This makes quinoa one of the best sources of plant protein. It also provides riboflavin (a B vitamin), vitamin E, iron, magnesium, potassium, zinc, and fiber. For more on quinoa, see Nutrition Note for Creamy Cranberry Quinoa (page 65).

ANALYSIS FOR 1 SERVING:
½ cup

Calories: 90, Fat: 1.8 g, Total carbohydrates: 16.5 g, Protein: 2.9 g,
Dietary fiber: 1.8 g, Sodium: 167 mg, Net carbs: 14.7 g, Carb Choice: 1

Sautéed Cabbage and Walnuts

Sautéing the cabbage in garlic gives it a refreshing bite, without the soggy, acrid consequences of traditional overboiling. Healthful walnuts add a nutritional and gastronomic bonus in this low-calorie, super low-carb dish, suitable as a side or a filling main course.

1 teaspoon extra-virgin olive oil
1 cup thinly sliced onion
½ cup thinly sliced red bell pepper
1 teaspoon minced garlic
8 cups ½-inch green cabbage pieces
½ teaspoon seasoned salt

½ teaspoon garlic and herb seasoning (salt-free)
1 cup water
½ cup chopped fresh parsley
¼ cup chopped walnuts

■ Heat the oil in a wok or large skillet over medium heat. Add the onion, bell pepper, and garlic and sauté, until tender, 4 to 5 minutes. Add the cabbage, seasonings, water, and parsley, and stir-fry until tender, about 5 minutes. Stir in the walnuts and serve.

► *Nutrition Note:* Cabbage has been a longstanding dietary staple for the human family for many thousands of years, with hundreds of varieties grown throughout the world. The main three types of cabbage found in American markets are green, red, and Savoy. Cabbage is rich in vitamin C, the B vitamin folate, potassium, and, like other members of the cruciferous vegetable family, it has an abundant array of potential cancer-fighting phytochemicals. Each type of cabbage has a unique nutritional profile. For example, red cabbage has more vitamin C than green, and Savoy contains more beta-carotene than other varieties.

ANALYSIS FOR 1 SERVING:
½ cup

Calories: 56, Fat: 3.3 g, Total carbohydrates: 6.4 g, Protein: 2.0 g,
Dietary fiber: 2.4 g, Sodium: 101 mg, Net carbs: 4 g, Carb Choice: free

---

Sautéed Spinach

Gently sautéed with garlic, red bell pepper, and onion, this very low-carb dish will make you (and spinach-promoting moms everywhere) happy.

1¼ pounds fresh spinach (about 20 cups)
¾ tablespoon extra-virgin olive oil
½ cup thinly sliced onion
½ cup thinly sliced red bell pepper

1 clove garlic, minced
1½ teaspoons garlic and herb seasoning (salt-free)
⅛ teaspoon salt

■ Wash the spinach and drain well. Heat the oil in a large skillet over medium heat. Add the onion, bell pepper, and garlic and sauté until tender, 4 to 5 minutes. Add the spinach, stir together, and cook until the spinach is wilted, 3 to 5 minutes. Mix in the seasonings and serve hot.

▶ *Nutrition Note:* Popeye was wrong! Spinach is not a good source of iron—nor calcium. While it does contain these minerals, spinach contains oxalic acid, too, which greatly limits how much of the minerals we can absorb. However, Popeye seems to have ignored all the other impressive nutritional benefits of spinach: riboflavin, vitamin B_6, vitamin C, vitamin K, folate, and magnesium. Spinach also abounds in the antioxidant carotenoids, beta-carotene, lutein, and xeaxanthin—all yellow-orange pigments. We don't see them because they're masked by the green pigment chlorophyll. Lutein and xeaxanthin are antioxidant soldiers in the macula of the eye, so spinach is one of the best foods to protect the eye from age-related macular degeneration. If that isn't enough, spinach also contains several other potent antioxidant phytochemicals. So, eat your spinach, even if it isn't for the reasons the Sailor Man said.

ANALYSIS FOR 1 SERVING:
1 cup

Calories: 70, Fat: 2.0g, Total carbohydrates: 10.8 g, Protein: 6.3 g,
Dietary fiber: 6.5 g, Sodium: 258 mg, Net carbs: 4.3 g, Carb Choice: free

---

Smashed Potatoes

Nothing says "comfort food" like mashed potatoes. Leaving the skins on in our yummy version of the American favorite makes this recipe pop with flecks of red color and a "comforting" chewy texture. After the potatoes have been boiled, use an old-fashioned potato masher to mash rather than whip, for the right "lumpy" texture.

6 cups quartered small red potatoes (with skin)

⅔ cup unsweetened soymilk

2 tablespoons Smart Balance Light Buttery Spread

1¼ teaspoons salt

■ In a medium saucepan, combine the potatoes with enough water to cover. Cook over medium heat until soft, 15 to 20 minutes. Drain. Add remaining ingredients and mash until chunky.

> **ANALYSIS FOR 1 SERVING:**
> ½ cup
>
> Calories: 136, Fat: 2.0 g, Total carbohydrates: 27.0 g, Protein: 3.2 g, Dietary fiber: 3.8 g, Sodium: 538 mg, Net carbs: 23.2 g, Carb Choices: 1½

Stir-Fried Vegetables

Fast, fresh, and jam-packed with wholesome vegetables, this colorful stir-fry is an ideal accompaniment to any Asian meal.

GLAZE FOR STIR-FRY

1 cup water

2 tablespoons Bragg Liquid Aminos

1½ teaspoons cornstarch

STIR-FRY VEGETABLES

3¾ teaspoons sesame oil

1¼ cups 1-inch yellow bell pepper squares

1¼ cups 1-inch green bell pepper squares

1¼ cups 1-inch red bell pepper squares

1 cup 1-inch red onion squares

2½ cups fresh quartered mushrooms

¼ cup 2-inch green onion lengths

3 cups diagonally sliced carrots

¾ cup canned baby corn

½ cup canned sliced water chestnuts

¾ cup canned straw mushrooms

2¼ cups broccoli florets

■ **Prepare the glaze:** In a small bowl, whisk together the water, Bragg Liquid Aminos, and cornstarch and set aside.

■ **Stir-fry the vegetables:** Heat the sesame oil in a large skillet or wok. Add the vegetables and stir-fry until mostly done, about 6 minutes. Pour the glaze over the vegetables and stir-fry another 2 minutes, until the sauce thickens and vegetables are crisp-tender. Serve immediately.

ANALYSIS FOR 1 SERVING:
1 cup

Calories: 82, Fat: 2.4 g, Total carbohydrates: 14.4 g, Protein: 3.2 g,
Dietary fiber: 3.9 g, Sodium: 223 mg, Net carbs: 10.5 g, Carb Choice: ⅔

Sweet Potato Fries

If you or your kids miss traditional French fries, we have the answer. Trade the unhealthy trans-fats and processed carbohydrates that bog down the fast food original, for a healthy boost of beta-carotene in this oven-baked, lower glycemic alternative lots of kids actually prefer.

3 cups ½-inch peeled sweet potato strips   ¼ teaspoon salt
Cooking spray

▪ Preheat the oven to 350°F. Spray a baking sheet with cooking spray. Spread the sweet potato on prepared baking sheet, and spray the sweet potato for 1 second. Sprinkle the salt over the sweet potato. Bake for 30 to 35 minutes, until tender, turning potatoes over halfway through baking time.

▸ *Nutrition Note:* Sweet potatoes are one of the most nutritious foods in the vegetable kingdom. They're low in fat, high in fiber, a good source of vitamin B_6, vitamin C, vitamin E, iron, and potassium. Their orange color comes from the immune-boosting, antioxidant phytochemical called beta-carotene. In fact, sweet potatoes boast more beta-carotene than any other vegetable, including carrots. If that isn't enough, sweet potatoes contain other phytochemicals that are potential cancer-fighters. See Nutrition Note for Baked Sweet Potato (page 176) to learn more about sweet potatoes.

ANALYSIS FOR 1 SERVING:
½ cup

Calories: 92, Fat: 0.2 g, Total carbohydrates: 21.4 g, Protein: 1.5 g,
Dietary fiber: 2.6 g, Sodium: 107 mg, Net carbs: 18.8 g, Carb Choice: 1

Pita Chips

*T*hese wholesome little triangles, perfect for dipping, satisfy the urge for a crunchy chip, which just doesn't go away once you get a diabetes diagnosis. But these chips are diabetic-friendly because they're made from low-glycemic, low-sodium whole grain Ezekiel 4:9 pocket bread. And they're oven-baked, not fried, so as long as you watch your portions, you can enjoy them with our Classic Hummus (page 217), Linda K.'s Low-Fat Faux Basil Pesto (page 221), Guacamole Rico (page 219), Spinach-Artichoke Dip (page 230), or anywhere a crunchy chip is called for.

1 Ezekiel 4:9 Prophet's pocket bread or
other whole wheat pita bread

Cooking spray

▪ Preheat the oven to 400°F. Cut pita pocket into 8 triangular-shaped pizza slices. Unfold each slice and tear in half. Place on an unsprayed baking sheet, and spray triangles for 2 seconds with cooking spray. Bake for 8 to 10 minutes, until crispy and brown.

▶ *Nutrition Note:* We especially like Ezekiel 4:9 pita bread because, besides being whole grain, it contains lentils and soy flour, both of which help regulate blood sugar.

ANALYSIS FOR 1 SERVING:
8 pita chips (½ pita pocket)

Calories: 62, Fat: 1.0 g, Total carbohydrates: 10.5 g, Protein: 3.6 g,
Dietary fiber: 2.3 g, Sodium: 60 mg, Net carbs: 8.2 g, Carb Choice: ½

Tortilla Strips

There's something ineffably enjoyable about crispy tortilla strips floating atop hot Southwest Soup (page 94).

1 Food for Life Sprouted Corn tortilla or   Cooking spray
  other corn tortilla

- Preheat the oven to 350°F. Cut the tortillas into quarters. Stack quarters and cut into ¼-inch strips (48 strips total). Place on an unsprayed baking sheet and spray with cooking spray for 1 second. Bake for 10 minutes.

ANALYSIS FOR 1 SERVING:
6 strips

Calories: 8, Fat: 0.2 g, Total carbohydrates: 1.6 g, Protein: 0.1 g,
Dietary fiber: 0.1 g, Sodium: 0 mg, Net carbs: 1.5 g, Carb Choice: free

---

Toasted Cashews

In our LCA kitchens, cashews are the base of some of our favorite recipes. It's not just that they're versatile and tasty, either. Since the 1990s, many thousands of people have been studied in five major studies that linked moderate nut consumption to lower risk of heart attack, and even reduced the risk of type-2 diabetes.

2 cups raw cashew pieces

■ Preheat the oven to 250°F. Spread the cashews on an unsprayed baking sheet and toast for 20 minutes, until lightly browned. Immediately remove from the baking sheet and cool before storing in the refrigerator in a covered container.

ANALYSIS FOR 1 SERVING:
2 tablespoons

Calories: 99, Fat: 8.2 g, Total carbohydrates: 5.1 g, Protein: 2.9 g,
Dietary fiber: 0.6 g, Sodium: 2 mg, Net carbohydrates: 4.5 g, Carb Choice: ½

Toasted Pecans

MAKES 1 CUP; 48 (1-TEASPOON) SERVINGS

Heart-healthy pecans are more than mere adornments to sweet confections. Thanks to their high monounsaturated fat content, they, along with almonds, are likely to help control blood sugar without raising cholesterol and triglycerides. Just remember to watch your portion size. A small toaster oven works well for toasting nuts.

1 cup chopped pecans

- Preheat the oven to 275°F. Spread the pecans on an unsprayed baking sheet and toast for 10 minutes, until lightly browned. Immediately remove from the baking sheet and cool before storing in a covered container in the refrigerator.

> **ANALYSIS FOR 1 SERVING:**
> 1 teaspoon
>
> Calories: 18, Fat: 1.9 g, Total carbohydrates: 0.3 g, Protein: 0.2 g,
> Dietary fiber: 0.2 g, Sodium: 0.2 mg, Net carbs: 0.1 g, Carb Choice: free

Toasted Walnuts

Probably more than any other nut, the humble walnut is a nutritional wunderkind.

1 cup chopped walnuts

■ Preheat the oven to 275°F. Spread the walnuts on an unsprayed baking sheet and toast for 10 minutes, until lightly browned. Immediately remove from the baking sheet and cool before storing in a covered container in the refrigerator.

▶ *Nutrition Note:* Need another reason to incorporate more walnuts into your diet? How about stronger bones? Research has found that foods high in omega-3 fatty acids (linolenic) can help maintain bone health. These fats reduce the activity of osteoclasts, cells that break down bones. Black and English walnuts are good sources of omega-3s, which come with none of the risk of toxic carcinogenic pesticides found in fish. In addition, walnuts are also high in tryptophan, necessary for the body to create serotonin and melatonin, which aid in proper sleep cycles. Their tryptophan content is also one reason walnuts are associated with big drops in cholesterol. See the Nutrition Note for Walnut Wheat Berries (page 72) to learn more about walnuts.

ANALYSIS FOR 1 SERVING:
1 tablespoon

Calories: 49, Fat: 4.9 g, Total carbohydrates: 1.0 g, Protein: 1.1 g,
Dietary fiber: 0.5 g, Sodium: 0 mg, Net carbs: 0.5 g, Carb Choice: free

---

SAUCES, SPREADS, AND DIPS

Sometimes the recipes in this section play a critical support-ing role—you wouldn't enjoy our Gourmet Eggplant Stacks (page 136) as much without our Chunky Marinara Sauce or our Savory Dinner Roast (page 157) without our Windcrest Country Gravy. And sometimes these recipes stand alone—our Chunky Chickpea Spread and Tofu Egg Salad create terrific sandwiches for everyday lunches and picnics. Some of these recipes form the foun-dation for more advanced recipes—our own so-called "mother sauces," such as our Low-Fat Tofu Sour Cream and Low-Fat Tofu Mayonnaise. There are dips here to accompany whole wheat chips and fresh vegetable crudités, and sauces and glazes to spice up what-ever's on the menu.

But it's when you add up all the little flavorful "extras" on your menu that you often start to see a lot of unnecessary fat and calories. We've worked hard to maintain flavor, texture, and aroma in these recipes, even while ensuring they work for people with diabetes and other health concerns. We've even offered lower-fat versions of high-fat favorites. Common-sense portions are all it will take to make sure you don't go overboard with our sauces, spreads, and dips. Most of these recipes will have little or no impact on your blood sugar if you stick to our recommended portion sizes. But if you're worried about fat and calories, try not to double or triple up on these recipes. For example, when eating our breakfast Fiesta Burrito (page 56), choose either our Salsa Fresca, Gaucamole Rico, or Low-Fat Tofu Sour Cream Supreme as a topping—not all three!

Aioli

If you love garlic, this low-fat, nondairy, no-egg aioli is unbeatable for flavor. This French and Spanish spread is traditionally used for spicing up sandwiches and vegetables. You can dollop it on our Gazpacho (page 88), spread it on our Grilled Portobello Mushrooms (page 138), or make one of our pita pizzas (pages 153–155), using it as sauce.

1 (12.3-ounce) carton Mori-Nu lite, extra-firm silken tofu
⅓ cup water
½ teaspoon salt

1½ teaspoons onion powder
2 cloves garlic, peeled
2 tablespoons canola oil
1 tablespoon fresh lemon juice

■ In a blender on high, blend all the ingredients together until creamy, 1 to 2 minutes. Transfer to a bowl, cover, and refrigerate until serving. Extra sauce will keep for up to 3 days in the refrigerator.

ANALYSIS FOR 1 SERVING:
2 tablespoons

Calories: 25, Fat: 1.9 g, Total carbohydrates: 0.6 g, Protein: 1.4 g,
Dietary fiber: 0.02 g, Sodium: 93 mg, Net carbs: 0.6 g, Carb Choice: free

---

Alfredo Sauce

*T*his piquant sauce, which has no dairy ingredients, gives a zing to our Zucchini Ribbons (page 126) and to our Pita Pizza with Alfredo Sauce (page 153), and you can use it on whole wheat pasta, too. It works well hot or cold. Cashews, or any nut, need to be thoroughly blended or your finished product will be gritty. Rub mixture between your fingers to feel for grit. Try this Alfredo Sauce over cooked spaghetti squash for a tasty and exciting change.

¾ cup raw cashew pieces

2 tablespoons pine nuts

¾ cup water

¼ cup fresh lemon juice

1¼ cups low-sodium canned white beans, drained

3 cloves garlic, peeled

2 tablespoons Red Star nutritional yeast flakes

1½ tablespoons salt

¼ cup finely chopped fresh parsley

■ In a blender on high, blend the cashews, pine nuts, water, and lemon juice until creamy and grit-free, 1 to 2 minutes. Add the remaining ingredients, except the parsley, and blend until creamy. Place in a small bowl and fold in the parsley. The sauce will keep in the refrigerator for up to 3 days.

ANALYSIS FOR 1 SERVING:
¼ cup

Calories: 95, Fat: 5.3 g, Total carbohydrates: 8.7 g, Protein: 4.8 g,
Dietary fiber: 1.4 g, Sodium: 250 mg, Net carbs: 6.8 g, Carb Choice: ½

Asian Glaze

This traditional sauce will add an authentic Asian flavor to our Tofoo Yung (page 165).

1 cup cold water

1 tablespoon low-sodium soy sauce

1 tablespoon cornstarch

■ Whisk all the ingredients together in a medium saucepan. Cook over medium heat, stirring frequently until thickened, 12 to 15 minutes.

ANALYSIS FOR 1 SERVING:
2 tablespoons

Calories: 4, Fat: 0 g, Total carbohydrates: 1 g, Protein: 0.10 g,
Dietary fiber: 0.02 g, Sodium: 62 mg, Net carbs: 0.98 g, Carb Choice: free

---

Cashew Jack Cheese Sauce

MAKES 2 CUPS; 8 (¼-CUP) SERVINGS

It's surprising that this creamy white sauce made from cashews and brown rice actually has a mildly cheesy flavor that is a great alternative to regular cheese sauce, which is full of saturated fat. This low-fat alternative is a nice accompaniment to our Black Bean Enchiladas (page 132), and Gourmet Eggplant Stacks (page 136), and you can use it anytime you hanker for cheese.

1¼ cups water

¼ cup raw cashew pieces

1 tablespoon Red Star nutritional yeast flakes

1 cup cooked brown rice (unsalted)

1 teaspoon salt

¼ teaspoon garlic powder

1 teaspoon onion powder

1½ tablespoons fresh lemon juice

- In a blender, blend all the ingredients on high until creamy and grit-free, 2 to 3 minutes.
- Transfer to a bowl, cover, and refrigerate until serving. Extra sauce will keep in the refrigerator for up to 3 days.

> ▶ *Nutrition Note:* These nuts are the seeds of the fruit of the cashew tree that is native to Africa and South America, but grown in tropical climates throughout the world. Most cashews in the United States are imported from India. Like most nuts, cashews provide some fiber, protein, B vitamins, vitamin E, and potassium. Also like most nuts, they are especially rich in fat, most of which is the "good" unsaturated, heart-healthy kind. Along with pine nuts, cashews are a richer source of iron and magnesium than most nuts. See Nutrition Note for Pimiento Cheese Sauce (page 228) to learn more about cashews.

ANALYSIS FOR ONE SERVING:
¼ cup

Calories: 57, Fat: 2.3 g, Total carbohydrates: 7.8 g, Protein: 2.1 g,
Dietary fiber: 0.9 g, Sodium: 298 mg, Net carbs: 6.9 g, Carb Choice: ½

Chiapas Salsa

*T*his simple recipe originated with Bonnie's friend Joanie, who showed her how her family made salsa every day in Chiapas, Mexico. You can use this salsa with whole-grain, low-fat baked chips, and over any of our Mexican dishes, such as our Fiesta Burrito (page 56), Sombrero Olé (page 158), Black Bean Enchilada (page 132), Haystacks (page 140), or Tac-Waffles (page 63)—and you can eat it liberally because it's low-fat and low-carb. This is a traditional "hot" Mexican salsa. If you don't like your salsa so spicy, cut the cooked chilies in half and remove the seeds before boiling.

2 large fresh tomatoes, whole and unpeeled

2 jalapeño chilies, whole, stems removed

2 tablespoons diced onion

2 tablespoons finely chopped fresh cilantro

¾ teaspoon salt

■ Place the tomatoes and jalapeño chilies in a medium saucepan. Cover with water and boil until soft, about 10 minutes. Drain. Place the tomatoes and chilies in a blender and blend well on high to the consistency of tomato sauce, about 1 minute. Pour into a small bowl and stir in the onion, cilantro, and salt. Extra sauce will keep in the refrigerator for up to 3 days.

▶ *Nutrition Note:* Chili peppers are low in fat, carbohydrate, protein, fiber, and calories, but are a good source of vitamin C and potassium. Like sweet peppers, the green chili peppers are mature, but will ripen and turn red if left on the vine (which makes them even hotter). Red chilies also contain more beta-carotene than their hot green cousins. The number of varieties of chilies is daunting, but a few of the most well known include Anaheims, cayennes, chipotles (dried, smoked jalapeños), and jalapeños. A chili's relative hotness is influenced by several things: maturity, soil, climate, and other conditions that all affect how much capsaicin is formed in the chili. This means that chilies on the same plant can have differing degrees of hotness. If you want to eliminate the heat, remove the seeds and ribs of the chilies. See Nutrition Note for Classic Hummus (page 217) to learn more about chilies.

ANALYSIS FOR 1 SERVING:
2 tablespoons

Calories: 7, Fat: 0.1 g, Total carbohydrates: 1.5 g, Protein: 0.3 g,
Dietary fiber: 0.4 g, Sodium: 129 mg, Net carbs: 1.1 g, Carb Choice: free

---

Chunky Chickpea Spread

This refreshing spread is a favorite with chicken- and tuna-salad lovers because it has a similar meaty taste with a cool, crunchy consistency, but without all the fat and calories.

4 cups low-sodium canned chickpeas, drained

1½ cups finely chopped celery

½ cup finely chopped red onion

½ teaspoon garlic powder

¾ cup Nayonaise spread, Tofutti Better Than Sour Cream, or Low-Fat Tofu Mayonnaise (page 223)

1 teaspoon celery salt, or to taste

2 tablespoons McKay's Chicken-Style Instant Broth and Seasoning, Vegan

■ Place the beans in a food processor and pulse a few times until they are chopped and chunky (no whole beans visible, but not mushy). Place in a bowl, add the remaining ingredients, and stir together well.

■ Transfer to a bowl, cover, and refrigerate until serving.

▶ *Nutrition Note:* Chickpeas, also called garbanzos, are a very versatile and nutritious bean with a mild meaty flavor. Like other beans, chickpeas are digested slowly, which promotes a gradual release of glucose into the bloodstream, making them an excellent low-glycemic food for helping regulate blood sugar.

ANALYSIS FOR 1 SERVING:
½ cup made with Nayonaise spread

Calories: 163, Fat: 6.0 g, Total carbohydrates: 22 g, Protein: 6.5 g,
Dietary fiber: 5.7 g, Sodium: 326 mg, Net carbs: 16.3 g, Carb Choice: 1

ANALYSIS FOR 1 SERVING:
½ cup made with Tofutti Better Than Sour Cream

Calories: 168, Fat: 4.9 g, Total carbohydrates: 26.2 g, Protein: 6.7 g,
Dietary fiber: 6.1 g, Sodium: 285 mg, Net carbs: 20.1, Carb Choice: 1⅓

ANALYSIS FOR 1 SERVING:
½ cup made with Low-Fat Tofu Mayonnaise

Calories: 134, Fat: 3.0 g, Total carbohydrates: 21.1 g, Protein: 7.0 g,
Dietary fiber: 5.5 g, Sodium: 245 mg, Net carbs: 14.1 g, Carb Choice: 1

Chunky Marinara Sauce

*T*his quick and easy marinara sauce is a staple in all our Italian dishes, such as Quick and Easy Eggplant (page 156), Gourmet Eggplant Stacks (page 136), Italian Stuffed Shells (page 141), and Spinach Lasagne (page 159). You can ladle it over our Nut Meatballs (page 148), or use it anytime you need a good homemade "gravy" (as the Italians say), but don't want all the sugar and salt of most jarred marinara sauces.

1½ teaspoons extra-virgin olive oil

1 cup chopped onion

2 cloves garlic, minced

2 (14.5-ounce) can diced canned tomatoes, with liquid (3 cups)

½ cup no-salt-added canned tomato sauce

1 teaspoon dried basil

½ teaspoon dried oregano leaves

½ teaspoon dried thyme

½ teaspoon salt

1 tablespoon fresh lemon juice

■ Heat the oil in a medium saucepan over medium heat. Add the onion and garlic and sauté, until tender, 3 to 4 minutes. Add the remaining ingredients and bring to a boil. Reduce the heat and simmer for 10 minutes.

▶ *Nutrition Note:* Tomatoes are famous for the pigment lycopene, which gives them their red color. In fact, tomatoes are the richest food source of health-promoting lycopene. More than 80 percent of lycopene in the American diet comes from tomatoes and tomato products. While we absorb lycopene from raw tomatoes, we absorb much more from cooked or processed tomatoes in the presence of a bit of fat. That makes marinara tomato sauce a nutritional hero. Lycopene is the powerful antioxidant carotenoid phytochemical that may help prevent prostate cancer, but it appears to protect against several other forms of cancer, too, as well as heart disease.

ANALYSIS FOR 1 SERVING:
½ cup

Calories: 39, Fat: 1.0 g, Total carbohydrates: 7.3, Protein: 1.3 g,
Dietary fiber: 1.6 g, Sodium: 286 g, Net carbs: 5.7 g, Carb Choice: ⅓

Classic Hummus

This traditional-style hummus, the best we've ever tasted, becomes very untraditional when we add the rich flavor of roasted green chilies. We serve it with our Pita Chips (page 204), and with fresh vegetable crudités. For your convenience, extra hummus freezes well. If you're not wild about chilies, you can substitute diced artichoke hearts, olives, red bell peppers, or any other vegetable.

2½ cups low-sodium canned garbanzo beans, drained

½ cup tahini (sesame seed paste)

6 tablespoons fresh lemon juice

½ cup water

4 cloves garlic, peeled

1 teaspoon salt (use half the salt if using regular canned garbanzos)

1½ teaspoons onion powder

1 (4.5-ounce) can chopped mild green chilies (½ cup)

■ Combine all the ingredients, except the chilies, in a blender, and blend on high until smooth and creamy, 1 to 2 minutes. Pour into a bowl and stir in the chilies. Cover and refrigerate until chilled before serving. Leftover hummus will keep in the refrigerator for up to 3 days.

▶ *Nutrition Note:* The hallmark of chili peppers is their fiery taste, which comes from a volatile phytochemical by the name of capsaicin. Capsaicin appears to have antioxidant, cancer-fighting, and heart-protective properties. Be warned, however, that capsaicin is so hot that a single drop diluted in 100,000 drops of water will actually blister your tongue. Surprisingly, chilies belong to the same genus as sweet peppers, *Capsicum*, the name obviously taken from the heat-generating compound, capsaicin. Sweet peppers are not hot, because they contain a recessive gene that just about eliminates the capsaicin. Besides their "fire," chili peppers tend to be longer and thinner than sweet peppers. See Nutrition Note for Chiapas Salsa (page 214) to learn more about chilies.

> **ANALYSIS FOR 1 SERVING:**
> ¼ cup hummus
>
> Calories: 146, Fat: 7.6 g, Total carbohydrates: 15.6 g, Protein: 5.9 g,
> Dietary fiber: 5.4 g, Sodium: 182 mg, Net carbs: 11.1 g, Carb Choice: ⅔

Garlic Tahini Sauce

This low-carb, pungent garlic sauce is a favorite served with our Baked Falafels (page 129). Depending on how much you use, the fresh garlic flavor can range anywhere from mild to eye-popping.

3 cloves garlic, minced

½ cup tahini (sesame seed paste)

¼ cup fresh lemon juice

2 tablespoons low-sodium soy sauce

▪ Combine all the ingredients in a small bowl and stir together well. Cover and refrigerate until serving. Store in the refrigerator in a covered container for up to 1 week.

ANALYSIS FOR 1 SERVING
1 tablespoon

Calories: 63, Fat: 5.4 g, Total carbohydrates: 2.9 g, Protein: 1.9 g,
Dietary fiber: 1.0 g, Sodium: 101 mg, Net carbs: 1.9 g, Carb Choice: free

---

Guacamole Rico

Smash ripe avocados into this lemony, buttery dip that no Mexican or Southwestern meal like our breakfast Fiesta Burrito (page 56) can do without. If you need to quickly ripen an avocado, place it in a brown paper bag with an apple. Once cut, avocados should be brushed with lemon or lime juice to prevent browning. When storing guacamole, you can place the pits on top of the dip, which also prevents browning. Discard pits before serving.

2 medium ripe avocados
½ teaspoon fresh lemon juice
½ teaspoon salt

¼ teaspoon garlic powder
¼ cup chopped onion
4½ teaspoons fresh chopped cilantro (optional)

■ Wash the avocados, then cut in half. Scoop the avocado flesh into a bowl and discard the skins and pits. Add the remaining ingredients and mash by hand, or pulse together on the low setting of a food processor if you like it chunky, or process longer for a smoother consistency. Transfer to a bowl and serve immediately or cover and refrigerate until serving.

▶ *Nutrition Note:* We like avocados because even though they're a high-fat tropical fruit, two-thirds of their fat is the good, monounsaturated kind that, when substituted for saturated fat, helps lower LDL (bad) cholesterol levels. Avocados provide respectable amounts of fiber, potassium, magnesium, iron, vitamin B_6, niacin, folate, vitamin E, and more vitamin C than oranges. They also contain a long list of phytochemicals with various disease-fighting, health-promoting properties. Included in this list is beta-carotene and lutein, a carotenoid phytochemical that is also found in the macula of the human retina. Lutein is believed to protect against age-related macular degeneration, a major cause of visual impairment in the United States. See Nutrition Note for Tomato, Cucumber, and Avocado Salad (page 119) to learn more about avocados.

ANALYSIS FOR 1 SERVING:
2 tablespoons without cilantro

Calories: 48, Fat: 4.4 g, Total carbohydrates: 2.5 g, Protein: 0.6 g,
Dietary fiber: 1.5 g, Sodium: 101 mg, Net carbs: 0.9 g, Carb Choice: free

---

LCA Basic Tofu Sour Cream

The lemon juice and hint of honey give this nondairy sour cream alternative that authentic sour tang. The blended tofu handles the "cream" part. You can use this recipe whenever sour cream is called for. You can also stir in chives and garlic and use it as a vegetable dip.

1 (12.3-ounce) carton Mori-Nu lite, firm silken tofu

¼ cup canola oil

3 tablespoons fresh lemon juice

½ teaspoon 100 percent natural floral honey

½ teaspoon salt

■ In a blender, blend all the ingredients on high until smooth and creamy, 1 to 2 minutes, stopping periodically to scrape the sides. Transfer to a bowl, cover, and refrigerate. Store in the refrigerator in a covered container for up to 1 week.

ANALYSIS FOR 1 SERVING:
2 tablespoons

Calories: 39, Fat: 3.6 g, Total carbohydrates: 0.6 g, Protein: 1.4 g,
Dietary fiber: 0.01 g, Sodium: 93 mg, Net carbs: 0.59 g, Carb Choice: free

---

Linda K.'s Low-Fat Faux Basil Pesto

MAKES 1½ CUPS; 12 (2-TABLESPOON) SERVINGS

This vibrant pesto has a crisp, clean taste when blended with the earthy flavor of pine nuts. It's low-fat because its base is Great Northern beans, not oil—not that anyone will ever know. You can use it on whole wheat pasta, or brush it on grilled vegetables.

1 cup packed fresh basil leaves (4 cups loose leaves)

1 cup chopped Roma tomatoes

2 cloves garlic

2 tablespoons pine nuts

2 tablespoons Soyco Rice Parmesan Alternative, Vegan, or other nondairy (no casein) Parmesan cheese alternative

1 tablespoon extra-virgin olive oil

1/16 teaspoon cayenne pepper

½ cup low-sodium canned Great Northern beans, drained

■ In a blender, blend all the ingredients on high until creamy, about 3 minutes. Transfer to a bowl, cover, and refrigerate until chilled. Leftover pesto freezes well.

ANALYSIS FOR 1 SERVING:
2 tablespoons

Calories: 39, Fat: 2.2 g, Total carbohydrates: 3.5 g, Protein: 2.0 g, Dietary fiber: 1.2 g, Sodium: 184 mg, Net carbs: 2.3 g, Carb Choice: free

---

Low-Fat Lifestyle Hummus

This hummus is a lower fat version of a high-fat favorite, thanks mostly to the use of white beans to replace half of the high-fat sesame tahini. We've put this one to extensive taste tests, and no one can tell the difference. Use this hummus as a sandwich spread, or as a dip for vegetables or our Pita Chips (page 204). You may use any other white bean such as navy or cannellini.

2½ cups low-sodium canned chickpeas, drained

¼ cup low-sodium canned Great Northern beans, drained

¼ cup tahini (sesame seed paste)

6 tablespoons fresh lemon juice

½ cup water

4 medium cloves garlic, or to taste, peeled

½ teaspoon salt

1½ teaspoons onion powder

1 teaspoon ground cumin (optional)

1 (4.5-ounce) can diced mild green chilies, drained (optional)

■ In a blender or food processor, blend all the ingredients, except the chilies, on high until smooth and creamy, 2 to 3 minutes. Transfer to a bowl and stir in the chilies (if using). Cover and refrigerate until serving. Leftover hummus freezes well.

ANALYSIS FOR 1 SERVING:
¼ cup

Calories: 116, Fat: 4.4 g, Total carbohydrates: 15.3 g, Protein: 5.3 g,
Dietary fiber: 4.2 g, Sodium: 182 mg, Net carbs: 11 g, Carb Choice: ⅔

Low-Fat Tofu Mayonnaise

MAKES 2 CUPS; 16 (2-TABLESPOON) SERVINGS

There's a little oil, but no eggs, and we've taken the fat as low as it can go in this lively soy mayo you can use as a sandwich spread, or in any recipe that uses mayo, such as our Caesar Salad Dressing (page 102).

1 (12.3-ounce) carton Mori-Nu lite, firm silken tofu
⅓ cup water
½ teaspoon salt

1½ teaspoons onion powder
⅛ teaspoon garlic powder
2 tablespoons canola oil
1 tablespoon fresh lemon juice

- In a blender, blend all the ingredients together on high until smooth and creamy, 1 to 2 minutes. Transfer to a bowl, cover, and refrigerate until serving. Store in the refrigerator in a covered container for up to 1 week.

  ▶ *Nutrition Note:* As in our Low-Fat Tofu Sour Cream (page 224), we decreased the fat in this recipe by adding water and cutting the oil in half, without killing the flavor or texture.

> **ANALYSIS FOR 1 SERVING:**
> 2 tablespoons
>
> Calories: 24, Fat: 1.9 g, Total carbohydrates: 0.5 g, Protein: 1.4 g, Dietary fiber: 0.02, Sodium: 93 mg, Net carbs: 0.48 g, Carb Choice: free

Low-Fat Tofu Sour Cream

In this low-fat tofu sour cream we have not sacrificed one bit of the tang or the texture.

1 (12.3-ounce) carton Mori-Nu lite, firm silken tofu
⅓ cup water
½ teaspoon salt
1½ teaspoons onion powder
⅛ teaspoon garlic powder
2 tablespoons canola oil
3 tablespoons fresh lemon juice

■ In a blender, blend all the ingredients on high until smooth and creamy, 1 to 2 minutes. Transfer to a bowl, cover, and refrigerate until serving. Store in the refrigerator in a covered container for up to 1 week.

▶ *Nutrition Note:* As in our Low-Fat Tofu Mayonnaise (page 223), we decreased the fat in this recipe by adding water and cutting the oil in half, without killing the flavor or mouth feel.

ANALYSIS FOR 1 SERVING:
2 tablespoons

Calories: 20, Fat: 1.5 g, Total carbohydrates: 0.5 g, Protein: 1.1 g,
Dietary fiber: 0.02 g, Sodium: 74 mg, Net carbs: 0.48 g, Carb Choice: free

---

Mustard Sauce

*P*ungent and oniony, our mustard sauce can be used as a sandwich spread, or as a marinade to spice up grilled vegetables. It's also the ideal glaze for Grilled Portobello Mushrooms (page 138).

½ teaspoon extra-virgin olive oil
2 green onions, minced
2 tablespoons prepared mustard

½ cup Nayonaise spread
¼ cup water
1 teaspoon cornstarch

■ Heat the oil in a small skillet over medium-low heat. Add the onions and sauté until tender, 3 to 4 minutes. In a small bowl, whisk the remaining ingredients together until blended, and add to the onions. Cook, stirring occasionally, until thick, 12 to 15 minutes. Serve warm.

ANALYSIS FOR 1 SERVING:
1 tablespoon

Calories: 29, Fat: 2.6 g, Total carbohydrates: 1.3 g, Protein: 0.4 g,
Dietary fiber: 0.2 g, Sodium: 105 mg, Net carbs: 1.1 g, Carb Choice: free

No-Mayo Tartar Sauce

This simple tartar sauce is exactly like the traditional one, except with soy mayonnaise instead of egg mayonnaise. It tastes great on our Crabby Cakes (page 134).

¼ cup Nayonaise spread

1½ tablespoons Mt. Olive No Sugar Added Sweet Relish or similar no-sugar-added relish

■ Mix ingredients together and serve.

ANALYSIS FOR 1 SERVING:
2 tablespoons

Calories: 16, Fat: 1.6 g, Total carbohydrates: 0.5 g, Protein: 0.1 g, Dietary fiber: 0.1 g, Sodium: 63 mg, Net carbs: 0.4 g, Carb Choice: free

---

On the "House" Black Bean Dip

MAKES 1¾ CUPS; 7 (¼-CUP) SERVINGS

This zesty, smoky dip keeps for more than a week in the fridge, and can be eaten on the go. Don't let the long list of ingredients daunt you; it's quick and easy. Use this dip for baked whole grain chips or our Pita Chips (page 204). The "House" in the name of this recipe, by the way, is coauthor Bonnie House. If you can't find chipotle peppers, canned mild green or jalapeño chilies will work, too.

2 tablespoons jarred sun-dried tomatoes in olive oil, drained

¾ cup chopped green bell pepper

¼ cup coarsely chopped onion

2 cloves garlic, minced

1 cup cooked black beans, no salt added, or 1 cup low-sodium canned black beans, drained

½ canned chipotle chili in adobo sauce

1 tablespoon fresh lime juice

1 tablespoon fresh lemon juice

½ teaspoon salt

½ teaspoon garlic powder

1 teaspoon dried oregano leaves

1 teaspoon ground cumin

2 tablespoons low-sodium vegetable broth or 2 tablespoons water

■ In a small skillet, cook the sun-dried tomatoes, pepper, onion, and garlic until tender, 5 to 8 minutes. Place the sautéed vegetables and the remaining ingredients in a blender, and blend on high speed until smooth and creamy, 1 to 2 minutes. Transfer to a bowl, cover, and refrigerate until serving.

ANALYSIS FOR 1 SERVING:
¼ cup

Calories: 48, Fat: 0.6 g, Total carbohydrates: 9.0 g, Protein: 2.6 g,
Dietary fiber: 2.1 g, Sodium: 207 mg, Net carbs: 6.9 g, Carb Choice: ½

Pimiento Cheese Sauce

This is not your usual cheese sauce! The base is blended cashews, and the cheese color comes from pimientos. Use this on our Whole Grain Corn Grits (page 73), Armenian Lentil-Stuffed Peppers (page 128), Pita Pizza with Refried Frijoles Negros (page 155), Tex-Mex Casserole (page 161) or for any recipe calling for cheese. Freeze in small batches to have on hand when making these recipes.

1 cup water

6 tablespoons raw cashew pieces

1 tablespoon tahini (sesame seed paste)

3 tablespoons Red Star nutritional yeast flakes

1¼ teaspoons salt

2 teaspoons onion powder

¼ teaspoon garlic powder

1 (4-ounce) jar pimientos, drained (½ cup)

2 tablespoons fresh lemon juice

■ In a blender, combine all the ingredients and blend on high until completely smooth and creamy, 1 to 2 minutes. Transfer to a bowl, cover, and refrigerate until serving.

▶ *Nutrition Note:* Cashews are kidney bean–shaped nuts that grow in a double shell, which hang off the ends of small fruits called cashew apples. Have you ever wondered why cashews are always sold out of their shell, unlike other nuts? It's because they are related to poison ivy. The shells contain a caustic oil that requires the nuts to be carefully extracted in order to avoid contamination with this oil.

ANALYSIS FOR 1 SERVING:
2 tablespoons

Calories: 33, Fat: 2.1 g, Total carbohydrates: 2.6 g, Protein: 1.9 g,
Dietary fiber: 0.7 g, Sodium: 188 mg, Net carbs: 1.9 g, Carb Choice: free

---

Salsa Fresca

In the 1990s, salsa shot past ketchup and became America's condiment of choice. Our salsa is a Southwestern variation with all fresh ingredients and just a hint of hot. A great salsa for Pita Chips (page 204), baked corn chips, or spooned over Mexican entrées like our Tex-Mex Casserole (page 161)—even over Traditional Scrambled Tofu (page 75). Our Salsa Fresca is a low-calorie and super low-fat favorite.

2 cups chopped fresh tomatoes
¾ teaspoon salt
½ cup chopped onion
¼ cup chopped fresh cilantro

½ teaspoon fresh lemon juice
¼ teaspoon garlic powder
½ medium jalapeño chili, seeds removed, minced

- Pulse the tomatoes in a food processor until finely chopped. Add the remaining ingredients, except the chili, and pulse several times until the mixture is well-blended, but still slightly chunky. Transfer to a bowl, fold in the chili, and serve. Store leftovers in a covered container in the refrigerator for up to 3 days.

ANALYSIS FOR 1 SERVING:
2 tablespoons

Calories: 7, Fat: 0.1 g, Total carbohydrates: 1.7 g, Protein: 0.3 g,
Dietary fiber: 0.4 g, Sodium: 113 mg, Net carbs: 1.3 g, Carb Choice: free

---

Spinach-Artichoke Dip

A healthy, happy way to dip our whole wheat Pita Chips (page 204) or crisp, fresh vegetables, our special take on Spinach-Artichoke Dip has no cheese and no dairy to fill it with unnecessary saturated fat, trans-fats, and calories. Instead, this low-fat dip's foundation is blended butter beans. This generous amount is just right for a small dinner party. You can use navy or Great Northern beans instead of butter beans in this recipe.

4 cups fresh spinach

2 cloves garlic, minced

1 (15-ounce) can regular-sodium butter beans, drained (1½ cups)

1 cup chopped green onions

2 tablespoons chopped fresh basil

3 tablespoons plus 1 teaspoon fresh lemon juice

1 tablespoon Red Star nutritional yeast flakes

1 teaspoon dried dill weed

1½ cups finely chopped canned artichoke hearts (not marinated)

■ Rinse the spinach and cook in a medium saucepan with no additional water until wilted, 2 to 3 minutes. Drain well. In a food processor, puree the spinach, garlic, beans, green onions, basil, lemon juice, yeast, and dill until very smooth, 1 to 2 minutes. Transfer to a bowl and fold in the artichoke hearts. Serve warm or chilled. Leftover dip freezes well.

ANALYSIS FOR 1 SERVING:
¼ cup

Calories: 44, Fat: 0.2 g, Total carbohydrates: 8.6 g, Protein: 3.3 g,
Dietary fiber: 3.3 g, Sodium: 117 mg, Net carbs: 5.3 g, Carb Choice: ⅓

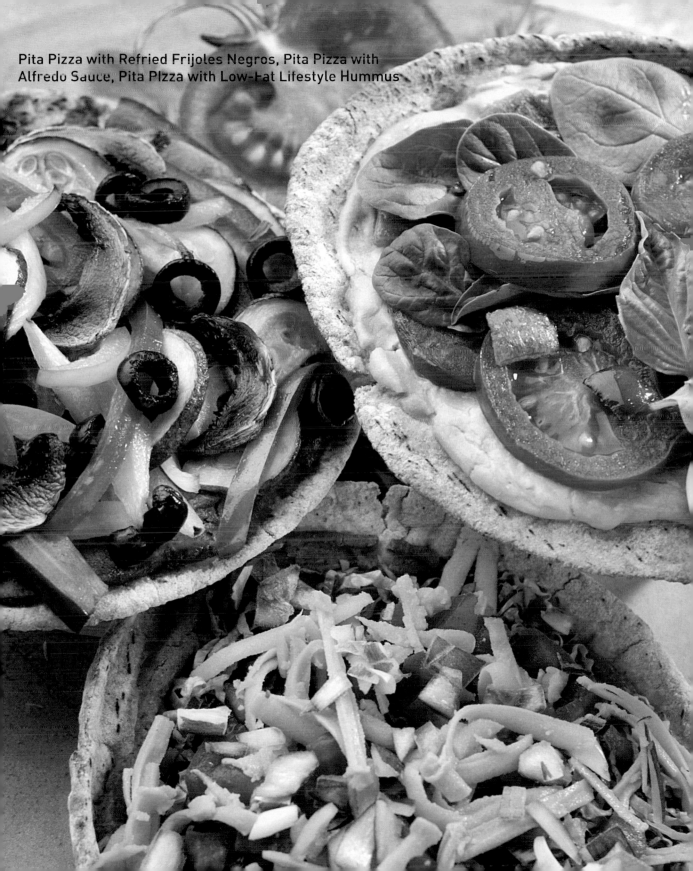

Pita Pizza with Refried Frijoles Negros, Pita Pizza with Alfredo Sauce, Pita Pizza with Low-Fat Lifestyle Hummus

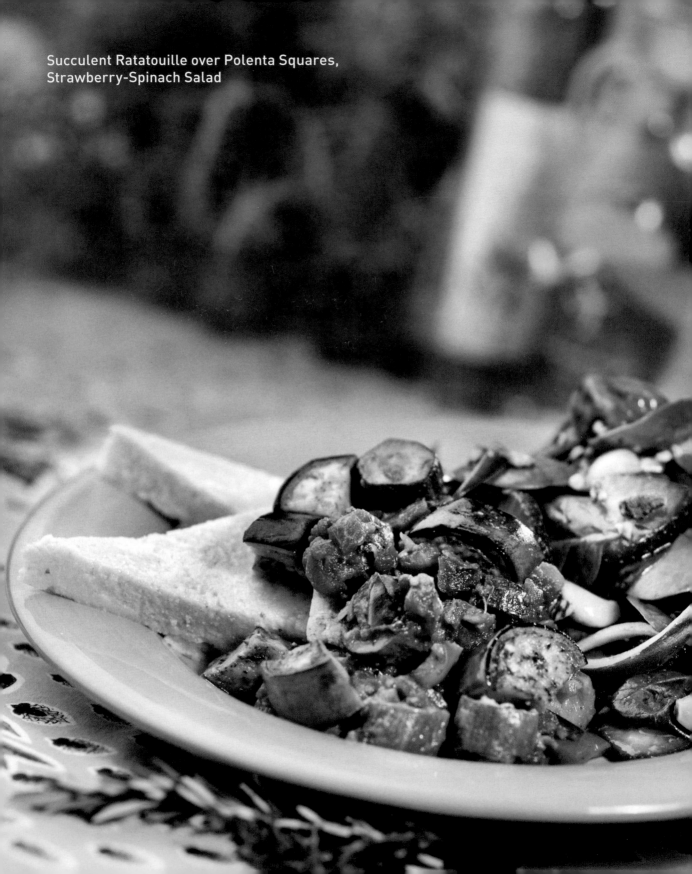

Succulent Ratatouille over Polenta Squares,
Strawberry-Spinach Salad

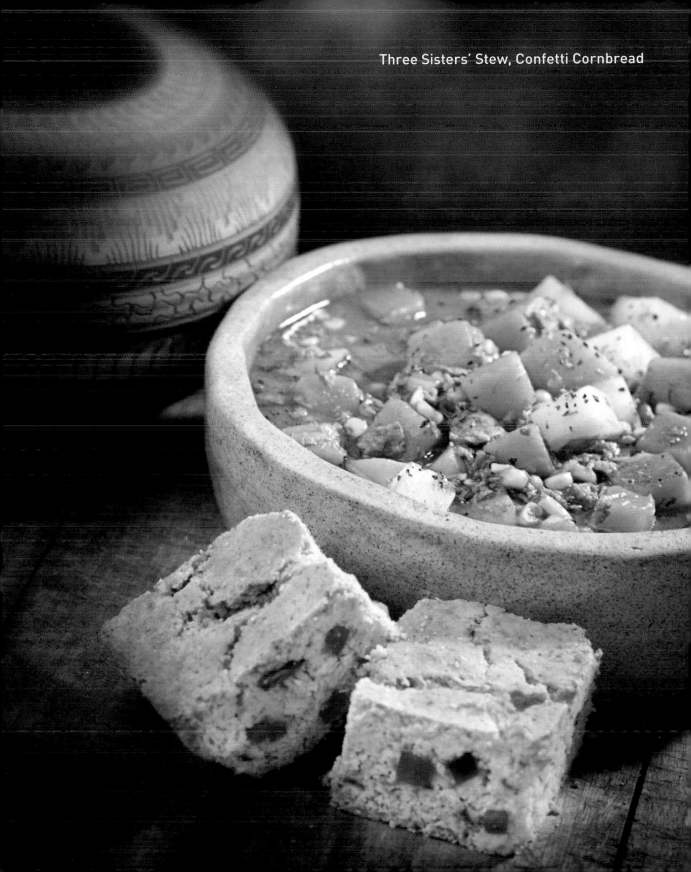
Three Sisters' Stew, Confetti Cornbread

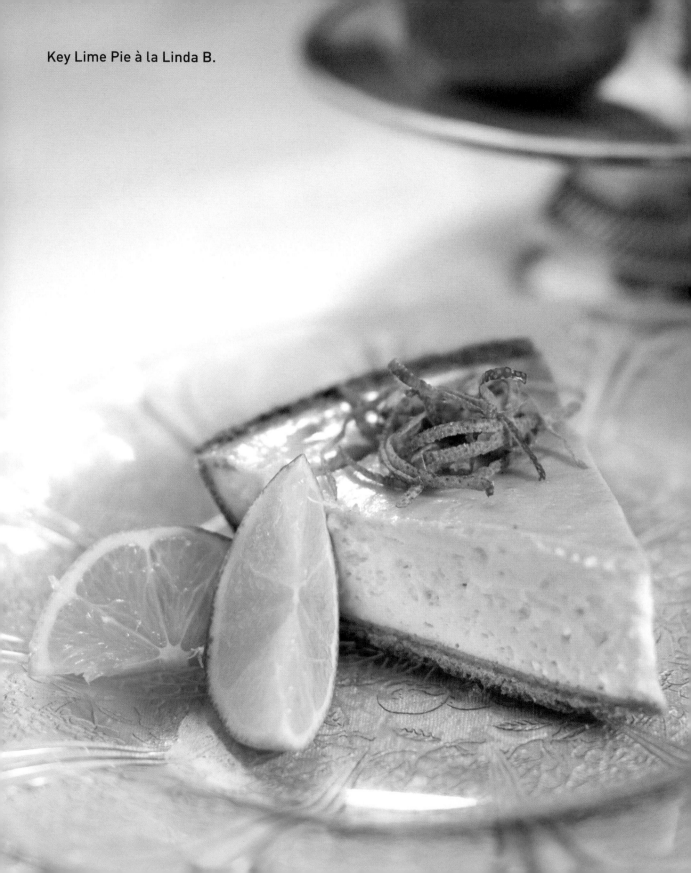

Key Lime Pie à la Linda B.

Sun-Dried Tomato Dip

MAKES 1½ CUPS; 6 (¼-CUP) SERVINGS

In this quick dip, the intense flavor of sun-dried tomatoes is further enhanced by citrus juice and light garlic. It may also be used as a sandwich spread, or as a pizza sauce.

½ cup jarred sun-dried tomatoes in olive oil (4 ounces), drained

1 cup Mori-Nu lite, firm silken tofu (8 ounces)

2 teaspoons fresh lemon or lime juice or 1 teaspoon each

¾ teaspoon dried thyme

⅛ teaspoon cayenne pepper, or to taste

½ teaspoon salt

2 cloves garlic, peeled

■ Place all the ingredients in a food processor and process until smooth, 1 to 2 minutes. Scrape the sides halfway through processing. Transfer to a bowl, cover, and refrigerate until serving. The dip will keep in the refrigerator for up to 3 days.

ANALYSIS FOR 1 SERVING:
¼ cup

Calories: 56, Fat: 3.0 g, Total carbohydrates: 5.3 g, Protein: 3.4 g,
Dietary fiber: 1.2 g, Sodium: 279 mg, Net carbs: 4.2 g, Carb Choice: free

---

Thai Peanut Sauce

This mildly sweet sauce has a bold peanut taste. It's awesome drizzled warm over our Linda B.'s Sesame Lettuce Wraps (page 146), or on our Stir-Fried Vegetables (page 202)—even over Mellow Brown Rice (page 194). The secret to keeping this recipe healthful and diabetic-friendly is to use natural peanut butter with no added sugar and no partially hydrogenated oil. The thickness of your peanut butter will determine the thickness of your peanut sauce. If you prefer some peanut chunks, use chunky peanut butter.

5 tablespoons creamy all-natural, no-sugar-added, nonhydrogenated peanut butter

3 tablespoons water

1 tablespoon low-sodium soy sauce

3 tablespoons fresh lime juice

2 teaspoons 100 percent natural floral honey

2 cloves garlic, peeled

1/16 teaspoon salt

1/16 teaspoon cayenne pepper

■ In a blender, blend all the ingredients on high until smooth and creamy, 1 to 2 minutes. Transfer to a bowl, cover, and refrigerate until using. Warm the sauce in a microwave before serving. Leftover sauce freezes well.

ANALYSIS FOR 1 SERVING:
1 tablespoon

Calories: 46, Fat: 3.4 g, Total carbohydrates: 2.8 g, Protein: 1.8 g, Dietary fiber: 0.4 g, Sodium: 89 mg, Net carbs: 2.4 g, Carb Choice: free

---

Tofu Cilantro Sour Cream

The subtle touch of cilantro, smooth texture, and zesty fresh lemon taste of this simple sour cream, will make you forget it's 100 percent dairy and guilt-free. This one's great on baked potatoes or as a vegetable dip.

1 (12.3-ounce) carton Mori-Nu lite, firm silken tofu

1½ tablespoons fresh lemon juice

2 tablespoons extra-virgin olive oil

1⅛ teaspoons salt

⅛ teaspoon cayenne pepper (optional)

1 small clove garlic, sliced

¼ cup chopped fresh cilantro

■ In a blender, blend all the ingredients on high until you no longer see specks of the green cilantro, 1 to 2 minutes. Transfer to a bowl, cover, and refrigerate until serving. Store in the refrigerator in a covered container for up to 1 week.

ANALYSIS FOR 1 SERVING:
2 tablespoons

Calories: 24, Fat: 1.9 g, Total carbohydrates: 0.6 g, Protein: 1.4 g, Dietary fiber: 0 g, Sodium: 185 mg, Net carbs: 0.6 g, Carb Choice: free

---

Tofu Egg Salad

This egg-free alternative to traditional egg salad rules the roost with all of the flavor of the original but no cholesterol. Some people think this spread tastes even better on the second day. If there is any left over, it will keep for up to 3 days in the refrigerator.

1½ cups Traditional Scrambled Tofu (page 75)

¼ cup plus 1 tablespoon Nayonaise spread

1 teaspoon prepared mustard

1 tablespoon plus 1 teaspoon Mt. Olive No Sugar Added Sweet Pickle Relish, other no-sugar-added relish, or ½ cup chopped celery

■ Combine all the ingredients in a bowl. Cover and refrigerate until serving.

ANALYSIS FOR 1 SERVING:
¼ cup with relish

Calories: 61, Fat: 4.4 g, Total carbohydrates: 3.0 g, Protein: 3.6 g, Dietary fiber: 0.6 g, Sodium: 196 mg, Net carbs: 2.4 g, Carb Choice: free

ANALYSIS FOR 1 SERVING:
¼ cup with celery

Calories: 55, Fat: 3.9 g, Total carbohydrates: 2.8 g, Protein: 3.2 g, Dietary fiber: 0.7 g, Sodium: 166 mg, Net carbs: 2.1 g, Carb Choice: free

---

Tofu Sour Cream Supreme

Our most popular soy sour cream goes great on a Fiesta Burrito (page 56) or any other Mexican or Southwestern favorite; just watch your portion size!

¼ cup Low-Fat Tofu Sour Cream (page 224)   ¼ cup Tofutti Better Than Sour Cream

■ Mix all ingredients together in a bowl, cover, and refrigerate until serving. Store in the refrigerator in a covered container for up to 1 week.

ANALYSIS FOR 1 SERVING:
1 tablespoon

Calories: 28, Fat: 2.0 g, Total carbohydrates: 2.4 g, Protein: 0.5 g, Dietary fiber: 0.3 g, Sodium: 59 mg, Net carbs: 2.1 g, Carb Choice: free

---

Walnut Hummus

Toasted walnuts and walnut oil give this hummus a powerful nutty flavor, which is softened by a trace of orange zest. Served with Pita Chips (page 204), this is an outstanding party dip.

⅓ cup walnut halves and pieces

1 clove garlic

2 cups regular-sodium canned garbanzo beans, drained

½ teaspoon grated orange zest

¼ cup unsweetened orange juice

2 teaspoons walnut oil

2 teaspoons sesame oil

¾ teaspoon salt

⅛ teaspoon cayenne pepper

■ Preheat the oven to 350°F. Spread the walnuts on an unsprayed baking sheet and toast for 8 minutes, until golden brown. Immediately remove from the baking sheet and cool. Put toasted walnuts in a food processor or blender with the remaining ingredients, and process until smooth, 3 to 4 minutes. Transfer to a bowl, cover, and refrigerate until using. Leftovers may be refrigerated for up to 5 days or frozen.

▶ *Nutrition Note:* See Nutrition Note for Walnut Wheat Berries (page 72) to learn about walnuts and the Nutrition Note for Chunky Chickpea Spread (page 215) to learn about chickpeas.

ANALYSIS FOR 1 SERVING:
2 tablespoons

Calories: 59, Fat: 3.0 g, Total carbohydrates: 6.4 g, Protein: 2.2 g,
Dietary fiber: 1.7 g, Sodium: 140 mg, Net carbs: 4.7 g, Carb Choice: ⅓

Windcrest Country Gravy

MAKES 2½ CUPS; 10 (¼-CUP) SERVINGS

*F*or some, mashed potatoes without gravy would be unthinkable. This is a meat-free, low-fat, low-carb, yummy brown sauce that complements any dish, like our Savory Dinner Roast (page 157), or Smashed Potatoes (page 201), or Cauliflower Mashed Potatoes (page 178) that cries out for gravy.

2¼ teaspoons McKay's Chicken-Style Instant Broth and Seasoning, Vegan

2¼ teaspoons McKay's Beef-Style Instant Broth and Seasoning, Vegan

1½ teaspoons extra-virgin olive oil

2¼ teaspoons Kitchen Bouquet or other liquid browning sauce

½ teaspoon garlic powder

½ teaspoon onion powder

1 tablespoon Red Star nutritional yeast flakes

½ teaspoon Bragg Liquid Aminos

2½ cups water

3½ tablespoons cornstarch

■ Combine all the ingredients, except ½ cup of the water and the cornstarch, in a medium saucepan, and bring to a boil. Whisk the ½ cup water and cornstarch together in a small bowl, add to the saucepan, and cook, stirring, until sauce returns to a boil and thickens, 12 to 15 minutes. Remove from heat and serve immediately.

ANALYSIS FOR 1 SERVING:
¼ cup

Calories: 27.7, Fat: 0.8 g, Total carbohydrates: 4.8 g, Protein: 0.8 g, Dietary fiber: 0.4 g, Sodium: 64.5 mg, Net carbs: 4.4 g, Carb Choice: free

---

AH, DESSERT. IF, like most of us, you're inclined to believe you deserve dessert once in a while, you should at least be sure you're not slowly killing yourself with the surfeit of saturated fat and calories, and the enormous spikes in your blood sugar associated with most desserts on the Standard American Diet. Enter the realm of *The 30-Day Diabetes Miracle* dessert menu. Years of research, experimentation, analysis, and taste-testing have culminated in this list. We don't just dupe you with a vague label of "sugar free," then pack in chemicals and harmful ingredients. True, there is no white sugar in any of these recipes; but there's also no high-glycemic white flour; no butter, no eggs, and no dairy, either. We think all our desserts taste terrific, but it's important to do a reality check. Until your taste buds adjust after a few weeks, it's possible that in some of these recipes you'll miss a few things you might have become accustomed to, namely the inimitable Twinkie-like taste and mouth feel of butter and partially hydrogenated oil. Just remember that if you or the person you're cooking for has diabetes or other chronic health concerns such as obesity and high cholesterol, you're also going to give chronic disease the miss by enjoying these delicious desserts in moderation.

There's something else we're proud of here. You'll notice there's no super-processed and possibly toxic chemical sweeteners like Splenda* (sucralose), Equal (aspartame/NutraSweet), and Sweet'N Low (saccharin) in any of our dessert recipes. That's very rare for a diabetic cookbook.

---

*There's actually one recipe ingredient in our book that contains a trace amount of Splenda: It's Mt. Olive sweet pickle relish, but the amount is so negligible, it's hardly worth mentioning.

Instead, we use mostly low-glycemic nonchemical sweeteners like fructose and floral honey (the kind made by bees, not factories). A few of our recipes use a small amount of organic cane juice, and one uses a small amount of organic brown sugar, and these can have a minor effect on your blood sugar. In general, though, your sweet tooth will be satisfied with our dessert menu, but your pancreas (or pump) will thank you for not taxing it with a need for tons of insulin. Your coronary arteries will thank you, too!

You'll also find no chocolate in our desserts, but don't despair just yet. If you'll pardon the pun, chocolate has a potential "dark side" we'd like you to consider. As any kid who's ever sneaked a bite of Mom's baking chocolate knows, chocolate's naturally bitter, so manufacturers add copious amounts of sugar for what they call "palatability." Sugar means blood sugar spikes, of course. What about sugar-free chocolate? Don't go there unless you can deal with the abdominal cramping (and worse!) caused by the sugar alcohols like maltitol used to replace the sugar. Also, more than half the calories in regular chocolate come from fat (specifically, cocoa butter), and a full two-thirds of that fat is the unhealthy saturated kind associated with serious chronic diseases like high cholesterol, obesity, heart disease, high blood pressure, and diabetes. Because an ounce of so-called healthier dark chocolate can contain a whopping 11 grams of fat, you'd need to cut that fat elsewhere in your diet to make room. Not to mention all those calories: It would take the average person more than an hour of intense exercise just to burn off the calories in a regular-size chocolate bar. And the anti-chocolate news gets worse. The confection's appeal goes beyond its deep brown hue and creamy texture. Chocolate contains psychoactive substances that stimulate the pleasure center of the brain, specifically the opiate receptors, contributing to its addictive quality. The term *chocoholic* is totally legit. In fact, chocolate's chemical actions go even further: It contains small amounts of methylxanthine stimulants, caffeine, and theobromine, which likely also contribute to its addictive nature. Chocolate also contains twelve different biogenic amines, which could potentially induce druglike neurophysiological effects, as well as fatty acids that may target the endogenous cannabinoid system of the brain. (That's the appetite-control center, by the way! The more you eat, the more you crave.) In short, chocolate's a sugar-filled, fat-laden, high-calorie, psychotropic *drug*. If you use it all, use it in moderation. Instead, enjoy our two fabulous alternatives, Diana's Delicious Un-Chocolate Brownies and I-Can't-Believe-It's-Not-Chocolate Cake.

Before you get baking and eating, we have five simple suggestions to stay healthy while enjoying these dessert recipes:

1. Don't hedonistically indulge in mass quantities of dessert: Stick to the portion sizes we recommend, and reserve dessert for special occasions and once or twice a week at most, not every meal or even every day.
2. On days you do eat a dessert, work its carb count into the daily total that's appropriate for you. This might mean skipping the side dish of potatoes in order to have a

cookie, or even skipping a meal on occasion. When it comes to dessert, don't *add it on*—*work it in.*

3. Give your taste buds time to adjust. It's possible that some people's first response to some of our desserts might be, "Wow, that's good, but it needs more fat." Ask yourself the question: Do *I* need any more fat? Really, give yourself time. It takes one a couple of weeks to adjust.

4. Consider what psychologist Douglas Lisle calls the "myth of moderation." Can you trust yourself to have a whole banana cream pie in the fridge, and only eat one-sixteenth of it twice a week? If you tend toward overdoing it with sweets, you should really think about trying to wean yourself entirely off. Otherwise you're in for torture.

5. Finally, have fun with these desserts: We've all made these pies, cakes, and cookies, and shared them with friends, family, and coworkers who'd previously challenged the concept of a plant-based diet, only to hear them rave, "Now *that's* a decadent cheesecake!" It's up to you whether to confess there are no unhealthy ingredients, or just say thank you and quietly smile, knowing you're helping your well-meaning critics stay healthy.

CHOOSING FRESH FRUITS

THE BEST DESSERT in the world is fresh fruit. Below are some hints about choosing fruits.

Apples

Taut skin, very firm when gently pressed. Avoid those with soft spots or punctures. Flavor and texture vary widely among varieties. Seek them out at local farm stands or farmers markets in the fall.

Bananas

In general, bananas are not diabetic-friendly, especially when they're ripe. However, if you want a banana, choose one that's plump, evenly colored, and green on the end.

Berries

Strawberries should be fragrant, shiny, firm, not too big, with healthy green stems. Blueberries should be firm, uniform in size, with no green or red areas. Raspberries should be full, just soft, but not oozing juice. Watch for mold and mush.

Grapefruit and oranges

Heavy for their size. With navel oranges; avoid severe bruises and soft spots. Juice oranges and grapefruits should be taut, with shiny skin.

Lemons and limes

Not much more than 3 inches from tip to stem, heavy for their size, with taut, thin skin, Avoid those with very hard skin. Should give slightly when pressed.

Melons

Not terribly diabetic-friendly, but if you choose one, be sure it's fragrant and heavy. Press end opposite stem to feel for a bit of give.

Pears

Fragrant, with no soft spots, punctures, or bruises. To eat right away, pears should give easily if pressed gently. Ripen quickly in a brown paper bag.

Stone fruits

Fragrant with taut skin. Avoid those with wrinkles and bruises. They should have some give when gently pressed. Handle carefully, and place no more than four per bag. Leave firmer fruit to ripen at room temperature.

Almond Fruit Cream

The almond extract adds an elegant flavor to this versatile fruit cream, which you can use as a pie topping, in fruit parfaits, or to spoon over berries.

1 cup slivered almonds

1 cup unsweetened pineapple juice

⅛ teaspoon salt

¼ teaspoon fresh lemon juice

½ teaspoon vanilla extract

½ teaspoon almond extract

2 tablespoons Resource ThickenUp or other instant food thickener

■ In a blender, blend all the ingredients, except the food thickener, on high until creamy, 1 to 2 minutes. Turn blender speed to low, remove the lid, and add the food thickener. Replace the lid, increase speed to high, and blend briefly until the mixture is thick. Transfer to a bowl, cover, and refrigerate until serving.

ANALYSIS FOR 1 SERVING:
2 tablespoons

Calories: 45, Fat: 3.2 g, Total carbohydrates: 3.4 g, Protein: 1.4 g,
Dietary fiber: 0.8 g, Sodium: 15 mg, Net carbs: 2.6 g, Carb Choice: free

---

Better Than Cream Cheese Frosting

Serve over Kennedy Carrot Cake (page 263), I-Can't-Believe-It's-Not-Chocolate Cake (page 265), or any cake or cupcake.

1 cup Mori-Nu lite, firm silken tofu (8 ounces)

1 cup Tofutti Better Than Cream Cheese, nonhydrogenated (yellow container, not blue)

6 tablespoons fructose

2 teaspoons vanilla extract

½ teaspoon fresh lemon juice

2 tablespoons Resource ThickenUp or other instant food thickener

¼ teaspoon salt

■ Process all the ingredients in a food processor until creamy, 2 to 3 minutes. Refrigerate in a covered container.

ANALYSIS FOR 1 SERVING:
1 tablespoon

Calories: 42, Fat: 1.8 g, Total carbohydrates: 5.9 g, Protein: 0.7 g, Dietary fiber: 0.3 g, Sodium: 62 mg, Net carbs: 5.6 g, Carb Choice: ⅓

Cashew Whipped Topping

*A*n adaptable, creamy topping for any pie or dessert, this recipe stands in nicely for whipped cream, with absolutely no dairy—and it stays fresh much longer in the fridge. You can use it as is, or add fruit, carob powder, or other flavorings in the final blend, depending on your tastes and recipe needs.

For a thicker topping that will stand up, increase the amount of instant food thickener to 3 tablespoons.

½ cup plus 2 tablespoons raw cashew pieces

1 cup plus 2 tablespoons water

2 tablespoons fructose

¼ teaspoon salt

½ teaspoon vanilla extract

2 tablespoons Resource ThickenUp or other instant food thickener

■ In a blender, blend the cashews and ½ cup plus 2 tablespoons water on high until you can rub the mixture between your fingers and not feel any grit, about 2 minutes. Reduce speed and add the fructose, salt, vanilla, and the remaining ½ cup water. Blend briefly on high, then add the food thickener, and blend for about 30 seconds. Transfer to a bowl, cover, and refrigerate until serving. Store in the refrigerator in a covered container for up to 1 week.

> **ANALYSIS FOR 1 SERVING:**
> 1 tablespoon
>
> Calories: 23, Fat: 1.5 g, Total carbohydrates: 2.1 g, Protein: 0.5 g, Dietary fiber: 0.1 g, Sodium: 22 mg, Net carbs: 2 g, Carb Choice: free

Easy Fruit Salad

This basic fruit salad is quick to make, colorful to look at, delicious to eat, and, thanks to the naturally low-glycemic properties of berries, diabetic-friendly. You can jazz it up with our Almond Fruit Cream (page 243), Sweet Summer Fruit Cream (page 271), or our favorite, which is listed below. When fresh berries are not in season, you can use frozen, unsweetened berries.

1 cup fresh blueberries

1 cup fresh raspberries

1 cup fresh sliced strawberries

6 tablespoons Tofu Whipped Topping (page 272)

■ Gently fold berries together in a bowl. Divide berries among 3 serving dishes and top each with 2 tablespoons of topping. Serve immediately.

▶ *Nutrition Note:* Besides all the health-promoting nutrients and phytochemicals in fresh berries, they are a wonderfully diabetic-friendly fruit because they're fiber-rich but not sugar concentrated, despite their sweetness.

ANALYSIS FOR 1 SERVING:
1 cup berries

Calories: 64, Fat: 0.6 g, Total carbohydrates: 15.5 g, Protein: 1.0 g,
Dietary fiber: 5.4 g, Sodium: 3.0 mg, Net carbs: 10.1 g, Carb Choice: ⅔

ANALYSIS FOR 1 SERVING:
1 cup berries with 2 tablespoons Tofu Whipped Topping

Calories: 70, Fat: 0.7 g, Total carbohydrates: 16.5 g, Protein: 1.0 g,
Dietary fiber: 5.4 g, Sodium: 18 mg, Net carbs: 11.1 g, Carb Choice: ⅔

Fancy Fruit Salad

This refreshing summer treat is simple to make, but tastes exotic and looks elegant. To add even more oomph to this fruit salad, add ½ teaspoon vanilla, banana, almond, coconut, or pineapple extract. If fresh pineapple is not available, use drained unsweetened canned pineapple chunks.

½ cup diced mixed apples (with peel)

½ cup sliced peeled kiwifruit

½ cup canned mandarin orange segments, drained

½ cup sliced fresh strawberries

½ cup cubed fresh pineapple

¼ cup Sweet Summer Fruit Cream (page 271)

■ Combine all ingredients in a bowl and stir together. Store leftovers in a covered container in the refrigerator.

ANALYSIS FOR 1 SERVING:
½ cup

Calories: 68, Fat: 1.9 g, Total carbohydrates: 12.6 g, Protein: 1.1 g, Dietary fiber: 2.0 g, Sodium: 10 g, Net carbs: 10.6 g, Carb Choice: ⅔

Fresh Fruit Sorbet

A blend of frozen bananas, berries, and stone fruits makes this brightly swirled dessert a favorite with ice cream lovers. Create your own specialty sorbet by using your favorite frozen fruits—we recommend low-glycemic temperate-climate fruits like cherries, berries, and peaches. Freeze bananas in a plastic bag until ready to use. If you have a Champion juicer, run the frozen fruit through the juicer, alternating handfuls. This will give the dish a beautiful rainbow effect.

4½ cups frozen bananas, cut into 3-inch chunks

5 cups frozen fruit of your choice (we like 2½ cups unsweetened frozen sliced peaches and 2½ cups frozen whole strawberries)

- Before preparing this dish, thaw all fruit for 30 minutes at room temperature. Process the fruit in a food processor for about 1 minute, stopping twice to break up clumps of frozen fruit. For soft-serve texture, serve immediately. For hard-serve consistency, freeze for 2 hours before serving. Scoop with an ice cream scoop into serving dishes.

ANALYSIS FOR 1 SERVING:
⅓ cup with ½ strawberries and ½ peaches

Calories: 52, Fat: 0.3 g, Total carbohydrates: 13.1 g, Protein: 0.73 g,
Dietary fiber: 2.1 g, Sodium: 2 mg, Net carbs: 11 g, Carb Choice: ⅔

Banana Cream Pie

MAKES 1 (9-INCH) PIE; 16 SERVINGS

The melt-in-your-mouth creamy consistency and sweet banana flavor of this decadent cream pie is a true miracle, considering it has zero dairy and is totally plant-based. It will make the end of any meal a treat.

1½ cups plain soymilk

1 tablespoon plus 1½ teaspoons Smart Balance Light Buttery Spread

¼ cup plus 2 teaspoons fructose

¼ cup water

⅓ cup Mori-Nu lite, firm silken tofu

¾ teaspoon vanilla extract

1½ teaspoons Vegenaise spread or Nayonaise spread

¼ teaspoon salt

⅓ cup plus 1 tablespoon cornstarch

¾ to 2 teaspoons banana extract, to taste

¼ teaspoon rum extract (optional)

1 cup sliced bananas

1 (9-inch) Arrowhead Mills graham cracker crust

■ Mix 1¼ cups of the soymilk, the spread, and ¼ cup fructose in a medium saucepan and bring to a boil. Blend the water, remaining ¼ cup soymilk, tofu, vanilla, Vegenaise, and salt in a blender on high until smooth and creamy, about 1 minute. Add the cornstarch and blend briefly. Add contents of the blender to the saucepan, and cook, whisking constantly, until thick and creamy, 5 to 6 minutes. Remove from heat. Fold in the 2 teaspoons fructose, banana extract, and rum extract (if using). Arrange the sliced bananas evenly on the bottom of the crust, and spread the filling over the bananas. Cover and refrigerate for 3 to 4 hours before serving. Refrigerate leftovers.

ANALYSIS FOR 1 SERVING:
1/16 of a 9-inch pie

Calories: 105, Fat: 3.8 g, Total carbohydrates: 16.4 g, Protein: 1.7 g,
Dietary fiber: 0.8 g, Sodium: 92 mg, Net carbs: 15.6 g, Carb Choice: 1

Cinnamon Secret Pie

Ready or not, here it comes—a bean-based pie! This all-time LCA favorite is a novel pumpkinless pumpkin pie alternative whose traditional spices and blended tofu and pinto-bean consistency make it smell, taste, and feel just like the original—only better and better for you. We nicknamed it "Two-Smile Pie," because your holiday guests will smile when they taste it, and again when you reveal the secret ingredient.

1 (15-ounce) can low-sodium pinto beans, drained (1½ cups)

⅔ cup 100 percent natural floral honey

1 teaspoon ground cinnamon

½ teaspoon ground ginger

½ teaspoon ground nutmeg

2 cups Mori-Nu lite, firm silken tofu

¼ teaspoon salt

1 teaspoon vanilla extract

1 tablespoon Ener-G Egg Replacer

1 (9-inch) Arrowhead Mills graham cracker crust

2 cups Tofu Whipped Topping (page 272)

■ Preheat the oven to 400°F. Combine all the ingredients, except the pie crust and the topping, in a blender and blend on high until completely smooth, 2 to 3 minutes. Pour into the pie crust and bake for 30 minutes. Cover the pie with foil, reduce the oven temperature to 350°F, and bake for 15 minutes. Cool. Cut into 16 slices and top each slice with 2 tablespoons of the topping. Refrigerate leftovers.

ANALYSIS FOR 1 SERVING:
1/16 of a 9-inch pie with 2 tablespoons Tofu Whipped Topping

Calories: 144, Fat: 3 g, Total carbohydrates: 25.7 g, Protein: 4.7 g,
Dietary fiber: 1.7 g, Sodium: 160 mg, Net carbs: 24 g, Carb Choice: 1½

Classic Lemon Pie

This is a quick and easy lemon pie with no egg meringue, and no lack of citrus bouquet or lavishly creamy consistency. If desired, top with Lemon Whipped Topping (page 255) or Cashew Whipped Topping (page 245).

2 cups unsweetened pineapple juice

⅓ cup 100 percent natural floral honey or fructose

¼ cup fresh lemon juice

½ teaspoon salt

1 cup unsweetened orange juice

7 tablespoons cornstarch

1 tablespoon grated lemon zest

1 (9-inch) Arrowhead Mills graham cracker crust

■ In a saucepan, bring the pineapple juice, honey, lemon juice, and salt to a boil. Combine the orange juice and cornstarch and whisk into the boiling mixture, and cook, whisking, until thickened. Stir in the lemon zest and pour into the pie crust. Refrigerate until chilled before serving. Refrigerate leftovers.

ANALYSIS FOR 1 SERVING:
¹⁄₁₆ of a 9-inch pie with no topping

Calories: 108, Fat: 2.6 g, Total carbohydrates: 21.4 g, Protein: 0.7 g, Dietary fiber: 0.5 g, Sodium: 103 mg, Net carbs: 20.9 g, Carb Choice: 1⅓

Holiday Pumpkin Pie

MAKES 1 (9-INCH) PIE; 16 SERVINGS

This traditional holiday pie uses tofu instead of eggs, but that affects only the cholesterol levels, not the flavor. Served with a dollop of Cashew Whipped Topping (page 245) or Tofu Whipped Topping (page 272), this pie is a richly flavored dairy-free marvel worthy of giving thanks and Thanksgiving.

⅓ cup 100 percent natural floral honey

3 tablespoons plus 1 teaspoon Sucanat organic brown sugar or other organic brown sugar

1½ cups Mori-Nu lite, firm silken tofu

1 cup plain, unsweetened canned pumpkin puree (we recommend Libby's brand)

⅛ teaspoon salt

1 to 1½ teaspoons pumpkin pie spice

1 (9-inch) Arrowhead Mills graham cracker crust

■ Preheat the oven to 400° F. In a blender, blend all the ingredients, except the pie crust, on medium until creamy, 1 to 2 minutes, stopping blender to stir contents. Pour into pie crust and bake for 30 minutes. Cover pie with foil, reduce oven temperature to 350°F, and bake for 35 minutes. Chill completely before serving, and top with your choice of toppings. Refrigerate leftovers.

ANALYSIS FOR 1 SERVING:
1⁄16 of a 9-inch pie with no topping

Calories: 93, Fat: 2.8 g, Total carbohydrates: 15.9 g, Protein: 2.1 g, Dietary fiber: 0.8 g, Sodium: 66 mg, Net carbs: 15.1 g, Carb Choice: 1

ANALYSIS FOR 1 SERVING:
1⁄16 of a 9-inch pie with 1 tablespoon Cashew Whipped Topping

Calories: 113, Fat: 4.3 g, Total carbohydrates: 17.3 g, Protein: 2.6 g, Dietary fiber: 0.9 g, Sodium: 88 mg, Net carbs: 16.4 g, Carb Choice: 1

ANALYSIS FOR 1 SERVING:
1⁄16 of a 9-inch pie with 2 tablespoons Tofu Whipped Topping

Calories: 112, Fat: 2.9 g, Total carbohydrates: 19.1 g, Protein: 3.2 g, Dietary fiber: 0.8 g, Sodium: 110 mg, Net carbs: 18.3 g, Carb Choice: 1

Just Plain Good Coconut Cream Pie

This exotic, tropical pie is delightfully light and creamy despite its total lack of dairy. Even seasoned cream pie lovers won't believe it's healthy. Create unlimited new versions of this versatile pie by omitting the coconut extract and adding pineapple, rum, or other flavored extracts.

¼ cup shredded unsweetened coconut

2¼ cups plain soymilk

⅓ cup plus 3 tablespoons fructose

2 tablespoons Smart Balance Light Buttery Spread

¼ cup water

¾ cup Mori-Nu lite, firm silken tofu

1 teaspoon vanilla extract

¼ teaspoon salt

1½ teaspoons Vegenaise spread or Low-Fat Tofu Mayonnaise (page 223)

½ cup cornstarch

1 to 2 teaspoons coconut extract, to taste

1 (9-inch) Arrowhead Mills graham cracker crust

■ Stir the coconut in a dry skillet over medium heat until golden brown, about 2 minutes. Immediately remove from pan, place in a small bowl, and set aside.

■ In a medium saucepan, bring 2 cups of the soymilk, ⅓ cup fructose, and the buttery spread to a boil. Place the water, remaining ¼ cup soymilk, tofu, vanilla, salt, 1 teaspoon fructose, and Vegenaise in a blender and blend on high until smooth, about 1 minute. Add the cornstarch and blend until mixed, about 15 seconds. Add contents of the blender to the saucepan and cook, whisking constantly, until thick and creamy. Remove from the heat. Fold in 2 tablespoons fructose and coconut extract. Spread into the crust and top with the toasted coconut. Refrigerate uncovered for at least 4 hours before serving. Refrigerate leftovers.

ANALYSIS FOR 1 SERVING:
1/16 of a 9-inch pie made with Vegenaise spread

Calories: 127, Fat: 4.9 g, Total carbohydrates: 18.4 g, Protein: 2.5 g,
Dietary fiber: 0.9 g, Sodium: 107 mg, Net carbs: 17.5 g, Carb Choice: 1

ANALYSIS FOR 1 SERVING:
1/16 of a pie made with Low-Fat Tofu Mayonnaise

Calories: 125, Fat 4.7 g, Total Carbohydrates: 18.3 g, Protein: 2.5 g,
Dietary fiber: 0.9 g, Sodium: 106 mg, Net carbs: 17.4 g, Carb Choice: 1

Key Lime Pie à la Linda B.

This pie offers a tart taste of the Keys with a luscious, pastel filling nestled in a graham cracker crust, all crowned with our Lemon Whipped Topping (opposite). Regular limes work well in a pinch, but for that really authentic taste, Key limes are the best.

2 cups Mori-Nu lite, firm silken tofu

½ cup Tofutti Better Than Cream Cheese, nonhydrogenated (yellow container, not blue)

½ cup fructose

2 tablespoons cornstarch

½ teaspoon vanilla extract

⅓ cup Key lime juice

2 teaspoons grated lime zest

1 (9-inch) Arrowhead Mills graham cracker crust

■ Preheat the oven to 350°F. In a blender, blend the tofu, cream cheese, fructose, cornstarch, vanilla, and lime juice on high until creamy, 1 to 2 minutes. Transfer to a bowl and stir in the lime zest. Pour into the crust and smooth the top with a rubber spatula. Bake for 30 minutes, until golden brown. Refrigerate uncovered until chilled before serving. Refrigerate leftovers.

> **ANALYSIS FOR 1 SERVING:**
> 1/16 of a 9-inch pie with no topping
>
> Calories: 117, Fat: 4.6 g, Total carbohydrates: 16.9 g, Protein: 2.6 g, Dietary fiber: 0.6 g, Sodium: 91 mg, Net carbs: 16.3 g, Carb Choice: 1
>
> **ANALYSIS FOR 1 SERVING:**
> 1/16 of a 9-inch pie with 1 tablespoon Lemon Whipped Topping
>
> Calories: 126, Fat: 4.7 g, Total carbohydrates: 18.1 g, Protein: 3.4 g, Dietary fiber: 0.6 g, Sodium: 113 mg, Net carbs: 17.5 g, Carb Choice: 1

Lemon Whipped Topping

This topping is light and fluffy with its spark of citrus, ideal for fruit or Key Lime Pie à la Linda B. (opposite).

1½ cups Mori-Nu lite, firm silken tofu	⅛ teaspoon salt
2 tablespoons fructose	3 tablespoons fresh lemon juice
1 teaspoon vanilla extract	⅛ teaspoon lemon extract

■ In a blender, blend all the ingredients on high until smooth and creamy, 1 to 2 minutes. Transfer to a bowl, cover, and refrigerate until serving. Store the topping in the refrigerator in a covered container for up to 1 week.

ANALYSIS FOR 1 SERVING:
1 tablespoon

Calories: 9, Fat: 0.1 g, Total carbohydrates: 1.2 g, Protein: 0.8 g,
Dietary fiber: 0 g, Sodium: 23 mg, Net carbs: 1.2 g, Carb Choice: free

---

Annie's Molasses Cookies

MAKES 32 COOKIES

A country kitchen on a crisp autumn day begs to be filled with the aroma of these fresh-baked cookies. Fill yours with the heavenly scent of cinnamon, cloves, and molasses, and the family will come calling for these scrumptious treats. These cookies can be baked and frozen for later use.

2¼ cups whole wheat pastry flour

2½ teaspoons Rumford baking powder

1 teaspoon ground cinnamon

1 teaspoon ground ginger

½ teaspoon ground cloves

¼ teaspoon salt

1 cup fructose plus 2 tablespoons for rolling

¾ cup Smart Balance Light Buttery Spread, at room temperature, or canola oil

¼ cup blackstrap molasses (do not use Grandma's or other light molasses or you won't get the right flavor)

3 tablespoons Ener-G Egg Replacer

4 tablespoons unsweetened or plain soymilk

■ Stir together the flour, baking powder, spices, salt, and 1 cup fructose in a bowl. In another bowl, with an electric mixer, beat the spread, molasses, egg replacer, and soymilk until creamy. Add the dry ingredients to the creamed mixture, and stir together. Cover the bowl and chill the dough for 20 minutes.

■ Preheat the oven to 350°F. Shape the dough into balls, using 2 tablespoons for each. Roll balls in the 2 tablespoons fructose. Place on an unsprayed baking sheet and bake for 16 minutes, until the centers are cooked firm and the tops of the cookies are cracked. Allow to cool on the baking sheet for 5 minutes before removing to a cooling rack.

ANALYSIS FOR 1 SERVING:
1 cookie

Calories: 84, Fat: 2.1 g, Total carbohydrates: 15.8 g, Protein: 1.2 g, Dietary fiber: 1.1 g, Sodium: 119 mg, Net carbs: 14.7 g, Carb Choice: 1

Oatmeal-Cranberry Cookies

MAKES 14 COOKIES

*W*hether you eat them from a brown paper bag or off a silver platter, cookies are a joy. But creating a healthy, diabetic-friendly cookie that still tastes good was quite a challenge for us, and took lots of experimentation and analysis. This cookie certainly meets the challenge, but remember, just one cookie is a serving (1 Carb Choice).

½ cup garbanzo flour
¼ cup whole wheat pastry flour
1½ cups old-fashioned rolled oats
¼ cup dried cranberries
¼ teaspoon salt
¼ teaspoon ground cinnamon

⅔ cup Smart Balance Light Buttery Spread, at room temperature
⅔ cup fructose
1 teaspoon vanilla extract
1½ teaspoons Ener-G Egg Replacer
3 tablespoons unsweetened or plain soymilk

■ Preheat the oven to 375°F. Spray a baking sheet with cooking spray. In a small bowl, stir together the flours, oats, cranberries, salt, and cinnamon and set aside. In a medium bowl, beat together the spread, fructose, and vanilla until combined. With a fork, whip the egg replacer and soymilk together until fluffy, and add to the fructose mixture. Add the dry ingredients and stir well. To make cookies, pack the dough into a 2-tablespoon measuring scoop, place on prepared baking sheet, and flatten slightly. Bake for 15 to 20 minutes, until lightly browned.

► *Nutrition Note:* When we think of cranberries we usually think of Thanksgiving—and combating urinary tract infections (UTIs). You already know about Thanksgiving, so here's more information on UTIs: A 10-ounce glass of cranberry juice is a well-accepted preventive strategy against UTIs, not just food quackery. How does it work? Cranberries contain a group of phytochemicals from the polyphenolic family, called "A-linked condensed tannins," which act like a protective coating, preventing E. coli bacteria from sticking to the walls of the bladder and urethra. The end result is that the bacteria pass right through the body without staying around to cause infections. The good news is that research has shown that dried cranberries are just as effective as cranberry juice. These same tannins may also offer protection against cancer and cardiovascular disease. Unfortunately, these same tannins that make cranberry juice so effective against UTIs taste sour. That's why most commercial cranberry products are heavily sweetened. However, this sour taste makes perfect sense from the point of view of the cranberry—it makes the tannins to ward off bugs. See Nutrition Note for Wheat Berry Waldorf Salad (page 120) to learn more about cranberries.

ANALYSIS FOR 1 SERVING:
1 cookie

Calories: 135, Fat: 4.8 g, Total carbohydrates: 20.8 g, Protein: 2.6 g, Dietary fiber: 1.7 g, Sodium: 111 mg, Net carbs: 19.1 g, Carb Choice: 1

Coconut Macaroons

These honey-sweetened golden bundles are our unique diabetic-friendly version of the sugar-laden Jewish original. The secret is that we replace a portion of the usual coconut with carrot, and use unsweetened coconut for the remainder. The result is a distinctive synthesis of Old World carrot cake and conventional almond-kissed coconut macaroons. Watch your portions, though, because even unsweetened coconut is still high in fat. These cookies can be baked and frozen for later use.

1 cup packed grated carrots
¼ cup water
½ cup 100 percent natural floral honey
1 teaspoon almond extract

2¼ cups shredded unsweetened coconut
½ cup whole wheat pastry flour
½ teaspoon salt

■ Preheat the oven to 350°F. Spray a baking sheet with cooking spray. Combine all the ingredients in a bowl and stir well. Let stand for 15 minutes. To make cookies, pack the mixture into a 2-tablespoon scoop measure and place on prepared baking sheet. Bake for 20 minutes, until golden brown. (Cookies will brown first on the bottom, so watch carefully!)

▶ *Nutrition Note:* Carrots are famous for being an outstanding source of beta-carotene, which provides the body with essential vitamin A, and functions as an antioxidant with several cancer fighting properties. In fact, carrots contain five of the six major carotenoids: alpha- and beta-carotene, lycopene, beta cryptoxanthin, and lutein. Research suggests that alpha-carotene, a close relative of the beta- variety, is more effective at stopping proliferation of human cancer cells than beta-carotene. If that isn't enough, carrots also contain a mix of several other cancer-fighting phytochemicals, including terpineol and apigenin. Carrots produce terpineol to fight fungi. Terpineol helps give carrots their down-to-earth flavor while helping fight cancer in our bodies. Apigenin has antibacterial, anti-inflammatory, antioxidant, and antitumor properties. Though carrots contain more sugar than most vegetables, you can eat them in moderation because their respectable fiber content helps prevent blood sugar spikes. See Nutrition Note for Kennedy Carrot Cake (page 264) to learn more about carrots.

> **ANALYSIS FOR 1 SERVING:**
> 1 cookie
>
> Calories: 84, Fat: 4.9 g, Total carbohydrates: 10.4 g, Protein: 1.0 g, Dietary fiber: 1.8 g, Sodium: 56 mg, Net carbs: 8.6 g, Carb Choice: ½

Peanut Butter–Flaxseed Cookies

Adding healthful flaxseed to good ol' natural peanut butter is an unusual twist to the all-American favorite, which takes these peanut butter cookies to new flavor heights—and lower fat depths.

½ cup Smart Balance Light Buttery Spread, at room temperature

¾ cup fructose

1 teaspoon vanilla extract

½ cup creamy, all-natural, no-sugar-added, nonhydrogenated peanut butter with salt

¼ cup Ground Flaxseed (page 64)

1½ cups whole wheat pastry flour

1 teaspoon Rumford baking powder

■ Preheat the oven to 325°F. In a medium bowl, beat the spread, fructose, vanilla, and peanut butter until creamy. In a small bowl, stir together the flaxseed, flour, and baking powder, and stir into the peanut butter mixture until well combined. To make the cookies, pack the dough into a 2-tablespoon measuring scoop, place on prepared baking sheet, and flatten the cookies slightly with a fork. Bake for 12 to 15 minutes, until golden brown. Immediately place on a cooling rack.

ANALYSIS FOR 1 SERVING:
1 cookie

Calories: 138, Fat: 6.7 g, Total carbohydrates: 17.5 g, Protein: 3.5 g, Dietary fiber: 2.1 g, Sodium: 119 mg, Net carbs: 15.4 g, Carb Choice: 1

Diana's Delicious Un-Chocolate Brownies

MAKES 16 (2-INCH) BROWNIES

Velvety, rich, moist, and nutty, these brownies are a sumptuous alternative to the usual suspects full of the sugar and saturated fat associated with their chocolate foundation. Here the fusion of coffee substitute, carob, maple, and vanilla flavors impersonates authentic chocolate taste without the guilt or addictive properties of the original. The organic brown sugar will add extra "chocolate" flavor.

1¼ cups whole wheat pastry flour

¼ cup Sucanat organic brown sugar, other organic brown sugar, or ¼ cup organic cane juice crystals

¼ teaspoon Rumford baking powder

½ teaspoon salt

½ cup Smart Balance Light Buttery Spread, slightly softened

¾ cup organic cane juice crystals

2 tablespoons Roma, Cafix, Pero, or other soy- and chicory-based caffeine-free coffee substitute

½ cup plus 2 tablespoons water

¾ cup Mori-Nu lite, firm silken tofu

6½ tablespoons Bob's Red Mill, Chatfields, or other brand carob powder

1 tablespoon vanilla extract

1 teaspoon maple flavoring

⅓ cup chopped walnuts

■ Preheat the oven to 350°F. Spray an 8-inch-square baking dish with cooking spray. In a small bowl, stir together the flour, sugar, baking powder, and salt. In a medium bowl, beat the spread and cane juice crystals with an electric mixer until creamy, 2 to 3 minutes. Stir the coffee substitute into the water and microwave until warm, about 30 seconds. Pour into a blender; add the tofu, carob powder, vanilla, and maple flavoring, and blend on high until creamy, about 1 minute. Add contents of the blender, the flour mixture, and nuts to the creamed mixture, and stir all together. Don't overmix. Spread evenly in prepared dish. Bake for 35 minutes, just until a wooden pick inserted in the center comes out clean. Cool before cutting into squares.

▶ *Nutrition Note:* Carob is that other dark brown powder from which many of the world's desserts derive. Carob comes without the negative health effects of the cocoa bean, from which chocolate is made. Carob powder is derived from the carob bean, aka St. John's bread or locust bean. Carob bean pods are long leatherlike pods that grow on a tropical tree. The tiny beans inside the pod are ground into carob gum (also called locust bean gum) and the pods are ground into carob powder, which is sold mostly in health food stores, either toasted or untoasted. While chocolate is naturally bitter, carob is naturally sweet. While chocolate is high in fat, carob is very low in fat. Carob does not contain caffeine or any other stimulants or psychoactive substances. But it is does contain some good stuff: fiber, magnesium, iron, and a surprising 100 milligrams of calcium in ¼ cup carob powder.

Warning: Be careful of various store-bought confections made with carob, as often manufacturers add fat and sugar. See the introduction to this chapter (page 239), and the Nutrition Note for I-Can't-Believe-It's-Not-Chocolate Cake (page 265), to learn more about chocolate and why we don't use it in our recipes.

ANALYSIS FOR 1 SERVING:
1 (2-inch) brownie

Calories: 134, Fat: 4.5 g, Total carbohydrates: 22.7 g, Protein: 2.5 g,
Dietary fiber: 2.5 g, Sodium: 141 mg, Net carbs: 20.2 g, Carb Choice: 1⅓

Kennedy Carrot Cake

MAKES 1 (13 × 9-INCH) CAKE; 24 SERVINGS

*O*ur guests say this lower fat, lower calorie version of the time-honored favorite really takes the cake. Because it has a bona fide vegetable in its name, carrot cake is shrouded in a kind of "health halo," despite the fact most recipes tip the scales at 500 or more calories and 30-plus grams of fat per slice. Our adaptation has the old-fashioned flavor, without the excess fat and calories.

½ cup Smart Balance Light Buttery Spread

1 cup fructose

1 cup grated unpeeled zucchini

¼ cup unsweetened pineapple juice

3 cups finely grated carrots

¼ cup shredded unsweetened coconut

½ cup water

2 teaspoons vanilla extract

½ cup dried cranberries

1 cup garbanzo flour

2 cups whole wheat pastry flour

2 tablespoons Rumford baking powder

¾ teaspoon salt

2 teaspoons ground cinnamon

½ cup chopped walnuts

1½ cups (24 tablespoons) Better Than Cream Cheese Frosting (page 244)

½ cup (24 teaspoons) Toasted Pecans (page 207)

■ Preheat the oven to 350°F. Spray a 13 × 9-inch baking dish with cooking spray. In a large bowl, mix together the spread, fructose, zucchini, and pineapple juice. Add the carrots, coconut, water, vanilla, and cranberries and mix well. In a separate bowl, combine the flours, baking powder, salt, and cinnamon. Gradually stir the dry ingredients and walnuts into the carrot mixture until well mixed. Pour into prepared pan, and put immediately into the oven. Bake for 45 minutes, or until a toothpick inserted into center comes out clean. Top each piece with 1 tablespoon of the frosting and 1 teaspoon of the pecans.

▶ *Nutrition Note:* When you think of carrots, you probably think orange. Interestingly, the early ancestors of the modern carrot were anything but orange—they were red, yellow, green, white, and purple. The development of the modern carrot took place around the 1700s, although why orange became its standard color is not clear. Carrots are a relative of parsley, dill, fennel, celery, and the wildflower Queen Anne's lace. Pull up a plant of Queen Anne's lace sometime and sniff the earthy roots, which smell just like carrots (some believe the modern carrot may be a domesticated version of it). Carrots are a low-calorie, low-fat vegetable, notable for fiber, potassium, iron, and vitamin B_6. Their nutritional trademark, though, is a mother lode of the orange pigment beta-carotene, of which they are the leading source in the American diet. In fact, the family of carotenoid pigments, of which beta-carotene is the most famous member, are named because they were first identified in carrots. Beta-carotene provides the body with the essential nutrient vitamin A. There's no danger of vitamin A toxicity from food sources with beta-carotene because the conversion of beta carotene to vitamin A is driven by the body's need for vitamin A. So what happens if you eat too many carrots? Nothing serious, though your skin might temporarily show a yellow-orange tinge from excessive beta-carotene intake, called carotenemia. See Nutrition Note for Coconut Macaroons (page 259) to learn more about carrots.

ANALYSIS FOR 1 SERVING:
1/24 of a 13 × 9-inch cake

Calories: 137, Fat: 4.4 g, Total carbohydrates: 23.4 g, Protein: 2.9 g,
Dietary fiber: 2.7 g, Sodium: 322 mg, Net carbs: 20.7 g, Carb Choice: 1⅓

ANALYSIS FOR 1 SERVING:
1/24 of a 13 × 9-inch cake with 1 tablespoon Better Than Cream Cheese
Frosting and 1 teaspoon Toasted Pecans

Calories: 197, Fat: 8.1 g, Total carbohydrates: 29.5 g, Protein: 3.9 g,
Dietary fiber: 3.2 g, Sodium: 384 mg, Net carbs: 26.3 g, Carb Choice: 1⅔

I-Can't-Believe-It's-Not-Chocolate Cake

MAKES 16 (2-INCH-SQUARE) PIECES

This is our plant-based, nondairy adaptation of a chocolate cake recipe from Country Living *magazine. The healthy substitutions we made don't affect its rich, moist chocolatey flavor. Wondering why anyone would present an Un-Chocolate cake? See the Nutrition Note below, and our note on chocolate in the introduction to this section.*

Important note: All ingredients must be at room temperature before making this cake.

1½ cups sifted whole wheat pastry flour

⅓ cup Bob's Red Mill, Chatfields, or other brand of carob powder

1 teaspoon Rumford baking powder

½ cup organic cane juice crystals or other nonliquid sweetener

¼ cup Sucanat organic brown sugar or other organic brown sugar

½ teaspoon salt

⅓ cup canola oil

1½ teaspoons vanilla extract

1 tablespoon fresh lemon juice

1 tablespoon Roma, Cafix, Pero, or other soy- and chicory-based caffeine-free coffee substitute stirred into 1 cup water and warmed in the microwave for about 30 seconds

■ Preheat the oven to 400°F. Spray an 8-inch-square baking dish with cooking spray. Stir together the pastry flour, carob powder, baking powder, cane juice crystals, sugar, and salt in a bowl.

■ In another bowl, combine the canola oil, vanilla, lemon juice, and coffee substitute. Pour liquid ingredients into the dry ingredients and stir together with a whisk until just barely mixed. Pour into prepared dish and put immediately on the center rack of the preheated oven. Bake for 25 minutes, until a wooden pick inserted into the center comes out clean. Cool before cutting into squares.

▶ *Nutrition Note:* Chocolate is nutritionally "hot" right now because of the discovery that it contains a class of powerful antioxidants called catechins, the same compounds that give tea its antioxidant clout. However, it's no surprise that chocolate contains antioxidants, because it's derived from a plant, and all plants have antioxidants. You don't need to eat chocolate to get antioxidants—just eat an abundance of plant foods. Try our cake and brownies made with the other tasty dark brown powder, carob: We think you'll be pleasantly surprised.

> **ANALYSIS FOR 1 SERVING:**
> 1 (2-inch) piece
>
> Calories: 119, Fat: 4.8 g, Total carbohydrates: 19.3 g, Protein: 1.6 g,
> Dietary fiber: 2.2 g, Sodium: 129 mg, Net carbs: 17.1 g, Carb Choice: 1

Peach Crisp with Cashew Whipped Topping

Bursting with natural sweetness and an unmistakable fragrance, rosy-skinned peaches are at the heart of this irresistible cobbler recipe, updated to exclude harmful ingredients, and ensure it's delicious yet still low-fat, low-calorie, and low-carb. As it bubbles to perfection in the oven, you'll remember why you love to cook—and why you love to eat dessert!

FILLING

4 cups frozen unsweetened peach slices

¼ cup fructose

1 tablespoon fresh lemon juice

1 tablespoon cornstarch

2 tablespoons water

CRUMBLE TOPPING

1½ cups old-fashioned rolled oats

2 tablespoons Smart Balance Light Buttery Spread

¾ teaspoon ground cinnamon

⅛ teaspoon salt

2 tablespoons fructose

¾ cup (12 tablespoons) Cashew Whipped Topping (page 245), to serve

■ Preheat the oven to 350°F.

■ **Make the filling:** Place the peaches, fructose, and lemon juice in a saucepan and bring to a boil. Whisk the cornstarch and water together, stir into the peach mixture, and cook, gently stirring, until the juice is thickened, 5 to 6 minutes. Pour the peach filling into an 8-inch-square baking dish.

■ **Make the topping:** Mix all topping ingredients together well. Crumble over the filling. Bake for 30 to 40 minutes, until golden brown. Top each serving with 1 tablespoon of Cashew Whipped Topping.

ANALYSIS FOR 1 SERVING:
¼ cup without topping

Calories: 94, Fat: 1.6 g, Total carbohydrates: 18.7 g, Protein: 2.0 g,
Dietary fiber: 2.2 g, Sodium: 42 mg, Net carbs: 16.5 g, Carb Choice: 1

ANALYSIS FOR 1 SERVING:
¼ cup with 1 tablespoon Cashew Whipped Topping

Calories: 116, Fat: 3.0 g, Total carbohydrates: 20.8 g, Protein: 2.5 g,
Dietary fiber: 2.4 g, Sodium: 63 mg, Net carbs: 18.4 g, Carb Choice: 1

Pumpkin Mousse Parfait

Layers of sweet, fluffy cashew, pumpkin, and pecans dazzle and delight. This recipe takes more prep time than most others, but when completed, makes a graceful presentation that your guests will tell you was worth the extra effort. Be sure you have a batch of chilled Cashew Whipped Topping (page 245) on hand.

1⅓ cups canned plain pumpkin puree, Libby's or other brand

⅓ cup fructose

½ teaspoon ground cinnamon

½ teaspoon ground coriander

½ teaspoon vanilla extract

¼ teaspoon salt

¾ cup Mori-Nu lite, firm silken tofu

¾ cup Cashew Whipped Topping (page 245)

2 tablespoons Toasted Pecans (page 207)

■ In a blender, blend all the ingredients, except the Cashew Whipped Topping and Toasted Pecans, on high until creamy, 1 to 2 minutes. Layer in 6 (6-ounce) clear parfait glasses or other glass dish as follows: 3 tablespoons pumpkin mixture topped with 1 tablespoon topping; repeat layers. Top each serving with 1 teaspoon of the pecans.

ANALYSIS FOR 1 SERVING:
1 parfait

Calories: 137, Fat: 5.2 g, Total carbohydrates: 20.1 g, Protein: 3.7 g, Dietary fiber: 2.1 g, Sodium: 169 mg, Net carbs: 18.0 mg, Carb Choice: 1

Raspberry Swirl Cheesecake

MAKES 1 (9-INCH) PIE; 16 SERVINGS

Everyone who eats this popular Windcrest Restaurant pie is shocked on two counts when you tell them its secrets. First, it has no dairy. Blended tofu and soy cream cheese is the secret to the perfect cheesecake consistency. Second, for a cheesecake, it's surprisingly low-fat, low-calorie, and low-carb. We strongly recommend using the nonhydrogenated version of Tofutti Better Than Cream Cheese, because it makes this pie come out perfectly smooth and creamy. The hydrogenated version of the cream cheese tends to make the consistency grainy.

¼ cup fresh or unsweetened frozen raspberries

2 cups Mori-Nu lite, firm silken tofu

½ cup Tofutti Better Than Cream Cheese, nonhydrogenated (yellow container, not blue)

½ cup fructose

2 tablespoons cornstarch

3 tablespoons fresh lemon juice (optional)

½ teaspoon vanilla extract

1 (9-inch) Arrowhead Mills graham cracker crust

■ Make a raspberry puree by blending the raspberries in a blender on high until smooth, about 1 minute. Press with a spatula through a small, finely meshed strainer into a bowl. Discard seeds. Set aside.

■ Preheat the oven to 350°F. In a blender (not a food processor or mixer) set on high, blend the tofu, Better Than Cream Cheese, fructose, cornstarch, lemon juice (if using), and vanilla until creamy, 1 to 2 minutes. Spread half of the mixture into the crust and smooth with a rubber spatula. Place half the raspberry puree in dollops on top of the filling. Using a wooden pick or a fork, swirl the raspberry puree into the filling. Top with remaining cheesecake mixture, smooth, and repeat procedure with remaining raspberry puree. Bake for 45 minutes, until the middle of the cheesecake is firm.

ANALYSIS FOR 1 SERVING:
1/16 of a 9-inch pie

Calories: 118, Fat: 4.6 g, Total carbohydrates: 17.2 g, Protein: 2.6 g, Dietary fiber: 0.9 g, Sodium: 90 mg, Net carbs: 16.3 g, Carb Choice: 1

Soy-Yogurt Berry Parfait

This parfait is simple, fast, stunning, yummy, and best of all, diabetic-friendly.

6 tablespoons Silk plain soy yogurt, or other brand plain soy yogurt

1 teaspoon fructose

2 tablespoons fresh or unsweetened frozen raspberries

2 tablespoons fresh or unsweetened frozen blueberries

2 tablespoons fresh or frozen unsweetened sliced strawberries

2 tablespoons chopped Toasted Walnuts (page 208)

In a small bowl, stir together the soy yogurt and fructose, and set aside. Gently toss the berries together. Layer in a parfait glass in the following order: 2 tablespoons mixed berries, 2 tablespoons soy yogurt, repeating twice more, and top with the walnuts.

► *Nutrition Note:* When choosing soy yogurt, make sure it has 12 grams of sugar or less per 1 cup serving.

> **ANALYSIS FOR 1 SERVING:**
> 1 parfait
>
> Calories: 120, Fat: 4.5 g, Total carbohydrates: 18.7 g, Protein: 3.1 g, Dietary fiber: 3.1 g, Sodium: 2 mg, Net carbs: 15.6 g, Carb Choice: 1

Spiced Poached Pears

This light and refined dessert with an exotic flair is ideal for entertaining in autumn or winter. Pears ripen from the inside out. Place unripened fruit in a brown paper bag and leave at room temperature to speed the ripening process.

4 firm pears (Seckel, Packham, Bartlett, Bosc, or a mixture)

¾ cup unsweetened apple juice (not concentrate)

1 teaspoon ground cardamom

⅛ teaspoon ground cloves

⅛ teaspoon ground ginger

⅛ teaspoon ground cinnamon

1 cup Cashew Whipped Topping (page 245)

8 teaspoons chopped Toasted Pecans (page 207)

■ Preheat the oven to 350°F. Peel and quarter the pears, discarding the cores. Slice each quarter in half lengthwise to make 8 slices per pear. Place the slices in an 8-inch-square baking dish.

■ In a small saucepan, heat the apple juice for 3 to 4 minutes, stir in the spices, and pour over the pears. Cover with foil and bake for 35 to 40 minutes, until the pears are tender when pierced with a knife. With a slotted spoon, remove the baked pears to individual serving bowls (4 slices or ½ pear per bowl), reserving the juices, and allow to cool to room temperature.

■ Pour the baking juices into a small saucepan, discarding the spice residue. Bring the juices to a boil and simmer uncovered until the juice is reduced to about ½ cup, about 40 minutes. Spoon 1 tablespoon of the reduced juice over each serving. Top each serving with 2 tablespoons of the topping and 1 teaspoon of the pecans.

ANALYSIS FOR 1 SERVING:
4 pear slices with 2 tablespoons Cashew Whipped Topping
and 1 teaspoon Toasted Pecans

Calories: 97, Fat: 4.9 g, Total carbohydrates: 13.3 g, Protein: 1.5 g,
Dietary fiber: 1.8 g, Sodium: 47 mg, Net carbs: 11.5 g, Carb Choice: ⅔

Sweet Summer Fruit Cream

Top a tantalizing fruit salad with this silky smooth nondairy nut cream. For a thinner consistency, use 1 tablespoon instant food thickener.

1 cup raw cashew pieces

1 cup unsweetened pineapple juice

3 tablespoons frozen apple juice
    concentrate

⅛ teaspoon salt

1 teaspoon fresh lemon juice

2 tablespoons Resource ThickenUp or
    other instant food thickener

■ In a blender, combine all the ingredients, except the instant food thickener, and blend on high until smooth and creamy, 1 to 2 minutes. Turn the blender to low, remove the lid, and add the food thickener. Replace the lid, increase speed to high, and blend briefly until mixture is thickened, about 20 to 30 seconds. Store in the refrigerator in a covered container for up to one week.

ANALYSIS FOR 1 SERVING:
2 tablespoons

Calories: 66, Fat: 4.1 g, Total carbohydrates: 6.6 g, Protein: 1.5 g,
Dietary fiber: 0.3 g, Sodium: 21 mg, Net carbs: 6.3 g, Carb Choice: ⅓

Tofu Whipped Topping

This lightly sweetened, fluffy topping adds the finishing touch when spooned over any of our delicious desserts. You can use it as is, or add fruit, carob powder, or other flavorings in the final blend, depending on your tastes and recipe needs.

1½ cups Mori-Nu lite, firm silken tofu
¼ cup fructose
1 cup water

1 teaspoon vanilla extract
¼ teaspoon salt
3 tablespoons Resource ThickenUp or other instant food thickener

■ In a blender, blend all the ingredients, except the food thickener, on high until smooth and creamy, about 1 minute. Turn the blender to low, remove the lid, and add the food thickener. Replace the lid, increase speed to high, and blend briefly until mixture is thickened, about 20 seconds.

ANALYSIS FOR 1 SERVING:
2 tablespoons

Calories: 19, Fat: 0.14 g, Total carbohydrates: 3.2 g, Protein: 1.1 g,
Dietary fiber: 0.01 g, Sodium: 44 mg, Net carbs: 3.19 g, Carb Choice: free

---

Upside-Down Apple-Oat Crunch

This quick and easy dessert does double duty as a sweet, healthy breakfast fruit dish. Try this recipe using Golden Delicious, McIntosh, Jonagold, Granny Smith, or Rome Beauty apples.

3 tablespoons old-fashioned rolled oats

1 tablespoon plus 1 teaspoon Smart Balance Light Buttery Spread, at room temperature

1¼ teaspoons fructose

¼ teaspoon ground cinnamon

2 teaspoons dried cranberries

2 medium apples of your choice

- Preheat the oven to 350°F. In a small bowl, mix together all the ingredients, except the apples. Layer the oat mixture on the bottom of an 8-inch-square baking dish. Cut the apples in half lengthwise and discard the cores. Place apples cut-side down on top of the oat mixture. Bake uncovered for 35 minutes.
- To serve: With a spatula, flip ½ apple along with ¼ of the crunch topping into a serving dish.

▶ *Nutrition Note:* Apples are one of the most common fruits, with about 7,500 varieties grown worldwide. They are a member of the rose family. While they contain some vitamin C and potassium, they're not particularly rich in other vitamins and minerals. Nor are they particularly noteworthy for plant pigments, aside from those in their skin. However, they are noteworthy for two important substances: fiber and quercetin. Apples abound in fiber, a full 80 percent of which is soluble fiber found in the white flesh. Most of the soluble fiber is pectin, known to lower cholesterol levels (and helpful in thickening jams and jellies). Most of the insoluble fiber, which aids in regularity, is found in the peel, which is also where the quercetin is concentrated. Quercetin is a powerful antioxidant with anti-inflammatory, anticancer, and heart-protective properties.

By the way, ever wonder why apples float? It's because 25 percent of their volume is air (not calories).

ANALYSIS FOR 1 SERVING:
½ apple with crunch topping

Calories: 80, Fat: 2.2 g, Total carbohydrates: 15.5 g, Protein: 0.8 g,
Dietary fiber: 2.4 g, Sodium: 28 mg, Net carbs: 13.1 g, Carb Choice: 1

Glossary of Unfamiliar Food Ingredients

THERE ARE SOME ingredients in our recipes that are quite familiar to plant-based cooks, but might remain a mystery to you until you transition. Unless otherwise specified, all of the items below can be found at well-stocked supermarkets (check the health food or organic sections) or health food stores. If you have trouble finding an item, contact the manufacturer via the Internet or go to www.diabetesmiracle.org, and we'll help you.

Almond milk. A milk made from almonds and water. Unsweetened almond milks are diabetic-friendly. Example: Blue Diamond's Almond Breeze.

Arrowhead Mills graham cracker crust. A graham cracker crust that is trans-fat-free, and partially whole grain.

Barley. Whole grain found as a whole kernel or flake. Pearl barley is not whole grain, but refined. Used as a breakfast cereal, in soups, or as a low-glycemic rice substitute in recipes.

Bragg Liquid Aminos. A nonfermented liquid bouillon made from soybeans and water, sometimes used in place of regular soy sauce.

Brown rice, Uncle Ben's converted. Available at any grocery store.

Buckwheat groats. Buckwheat is not a true grain, but the fruit of a leafy plant in the same botanical family as sorrel and rhubarb. Delicious as a low-glycemic, whole grain breakfast cereal.

Bulgur and cracked wheat. Bulgur wheat has been steamed, dried, and cracked into small gritlike pieces. Cracked wheat is cracked but not steamed.

Carob powder. Made from the locust pod, carob powder has a fat content of 2 percent, contrasted to chocolate's 52 percent. It's high in calcium, phosphorus, potassium, iron, and magnesium. Carob contains no tannin, caffeine, theobromine, or other psychoactive chemicals. May be used in place of chocolate.

Cheese substitutes. Nondairy (soy-based) alternatives made by Soyco, Vegan Gourmet (Follow Your Heart), Tofutti, Galaxy Nutritional Foods, and Soya Kass. Comes in most popular cheese flavors and forms.

Cilantro. Herb found in the produce section of most grocery stores and used in Tex-Mex cooking. Best when used fresh, as dry has very little flavor.

Citric acid. An organic acid found in food. May be purchased as a powder from your drugstore or in the canning section of most supermarkets. It's used in very small amounts to give dishes a lemony, vinegary tang. In most recipes you could crush a vitamin C tablet if you don't have citric acid.

Coconut milk, lite. This low-carb but still relatively high-fat product can be found in the Asian food section of most well-stocked supermarkets.

Coffee substitute. Instant hot drink powder made from roasted grains and chicory. Brands include Roma, Caffix, and Pero.

Edamame. Fresh green tender soybeans, often called "soy limas." Delicious steamed and used as a side to a hot meal or served cold in salads.

Ener-G Egg Replacer. A nondairy powdered leavening and binding agent used as a substitute for eggs in baked goods.

Ezekiel 4:9/Food for Life Breads. Diabetic-friendly breads and other products made from sprouted grains and beans, containing no flour. Tortillas (corn and wheat), pita breads, English muffins, and hamburger buns can all be purchased through the Food for Life bakery. Look for them in the cooler or freezer section of your health food store or some supermarkets.

Flaxseed. These golden or brown seeds are a good source of omega-3 fatty acids and fiber. Sprinkle a tablespoon of ground seeds on cereal, salads, or put in shakes. Soaked seeds make a good egg replacer in some recipes. See Ground Flaxseed (page 64).

Fructose. A simple, lower glycemic sugar to be used in place of regular sugar (sucrose).

Garbanzo flour. Flour made from cooked, dried, and ground garbanzo beans and often used in gluten-free baking.

Gluten flour. Made from the glutinous part of the grain, derived from whole wheat, that causes bread to be light and elastic. It's high in protein and helpful as a binder in some recipes.

Good Seasons Italian dressing dry mix. Available at any grocery store.

Kamut flakes. A whole grain flaked cereal available in most health food stores. There are several manufacturers, but we like Arrowhead Mills.

Kavli thin crispbread. Whole grain cracker made from whole rye flour.

Kitchen Bouquet. A rich, concentrated, and aromatic liquid browning seasoning and starter for making sauces and gravies.

Lentils. A small, tasty legume that does not need soaking, and has a full robust flavor. Even though there are more than 52 varieties of lentils, in this country green and red lentils are most often used.

Liquid Smoke. A liquid seasoning that adds a hickory-smoked flavor to recipes.

Masa harina. Finely ground whole grain corn used for making corn tortillas. Look for this item in the section of your grocery store that carries Mexican foods.

McKay's Beef-Style and Chicken-Style Instant Broth and Seasoning, Vegan. Powdered seasoning containing no animal fat or monosodium glutamate (MSG), used in place of chicken or beef bouillon. You can find this at well-stocked health food stores, or buy it in bulk from our website, www.diabetesmiracle.org.

Meat analogues. Veggie burgers (Boca Vegan Meatless Burger, Morningstar Farms Vegan Burger), sandwich meats, Morningstar Farms Griller Recipe Crumbles, Boca Garden Burger, Yves Veggie Bologna, and Morningstar Farms Chik'n Strips are all meat substitutes and are made from soy and gluten. Use in place of meat in recipes. Most grocery and health food stores have a large variety to choose from.

Nayonaise. A soy-based alternative to mayonnaise. Use on sandwiches and salads. We prefer this brand to Vegenaise, as it contains about half the fat. It's made by the Nasoya company.

Newman's Own dressings. Available at any grocery store.

Nutritional yeast flakes (Red Star). Yeast is a microorganism that belongs to the same family as edible mushrooms and other beneficial organisms used for medical and veterinary use. Red Star nutritional yeast is grown specifically for its nutritive value. An excellent source of protein, rich in vitamins, especially the B-complex vitamins, and an excellent source of folic acid. Their nutritional yeast is not made from the by-products of breweries, distilleries, or paper mills. It's not a genetically modified organism (GMO). It contains no added sugars or preservatives. Best when stored in a cool, dry place. Adds a mild, cheesy flavor to food.

Organic cane juice crystals. Granulated sugar from the evaporated juice of sugar cane. Florida Crystals Natural Sugar is one brand.

Pickles. Mt. Olive is a sweet pickle relish with no sugar. This is the only item in our recipes that contains a negligible amount of Splenda.

Pine nuts. Sometimes called pignoli seeds, they come from various types of pine trees, which grow around the world. Seeds come from the pinecones.

Polenta. Thick cornmeal mush that has set, so that it can be cut and sautéed or baked.

Quinoa. Not a true grain, but it looks like one, and is similar in use. It's related to leafy vegetables like Swiss chard and spinach. One of the best sources of plant protein. It's coated with a bitter resin (saponin), which should be rinsed off before cooking.

Rice milk. A liquid made from rice and used as a milk substitute. Brands include Hain Celestial Rice Dream. Beware that most rice milk is high glycemic.

Silk soy yogurt. A dairy-free yogurt alternative.

Rumford baking powder. Aluminum-free baking powder.

Smart Balance Light Buttery Spread. A nonhydrogenated, plant-based, buttery spread that has half the fat of other plant-based margarines.

Soybeans. A small, round cream-colored bean cooked, and eaten whole or used to make several alternative foods such as tofu and soymilk.

Soymilk. A liquid made from soybeans and used as a milk substitute. There are many brands, but we prefer Silk unsweetened (green container) as it is very low-carb.

Steel-cut oats. Usually imported from Ireland or Scotland. Made by thinly slicing oats lengthwise. They make a wonderfully chewy hot breakfast cereal that is low-glycemic.

Sucanat. Sucanat is dehydrated, freshly squeezed sugar cane juice. Wholesome Sweeteners makes this product, as well as other organic, unprocessed brown-sugar substitutes like Turbinado and Muscovado.

Tahini. A seed butter made from ground sesame seeds with a creamy consistency like peanut butter.

ThickenUp Instant Food Thickener (Resource [Novartis]). A commercially prepared starch that thickens liquids just by whisking (it doesn't require heating like cornstarch). You can find this thickener at some health food stores, or in the pharmacy section of most drugstores. If you don't see it on the shelf, ask for your drugstore to order some; Thicket, and Thicken are other examples.

Tofu. A curd made from blending, straining, cooking, and pressing soybeans. Because there are several kinds of tofu, read your recipe to see which one you need to use for the best results. Tofu has a fresh, clean odor with a creamy white appearance. Tofu that has spoiled is slimy to the touch, pinkish in color, and smells bad. We use two main types of tofu:

> **Mori-Nu lite, firm silken tofu.** This tofu comes in a 12.3-ounce carton that doesn't need to be refrigerated until opened. Used in creams, puddings, dressings, and sauces. This tofu comes in various consistencies, but we use firm in all our recipes.
> **Water-packed tofu.** Comes in a block surrounded by water, and has a slightly granular texture. Water-packed tofu needs to be refrigerated whether open or not. Use for scrambled tofu, fillets, or anywhere you want a cubed or crumbled consistency. There are different textures from soft and firm to extra-firm. Tofu can be frozen, but its consistency changes and becomes very spongy and chewy.

Tofutti Better Than Cream Cheese. A soy alternative to dairy-based cream cheese. It's cholesterol-free and lower in saturated fat than regular cream cheese, and tastes the same. We recommend only the nonhydrogenated version, in the yellow (not the blue) container.

Tofutti Better Than Sour Cream. A soy alternative to dairy-based sour cream. It's cholesterol-free and lower in saturated fat than regular sour cream, and tastes the same.

Tomato sauce, Hunt's no added salt. Available at any grocery store.

Vegenaise. A soy-based, cholesterol-free alternative to mayonnaise. Use on sandwiches and in salads. Contains less saturated fat than egg- and dairy-based mayonnaise. Made by Follow Your Heart.

Wheat berries. The seed or kernel of wheat. Most commonly ground into flour to make bread products. When cooked, it can be added to salads or loaves for a chewy consistency. Makes a delicious, low-glycemic, hot breakfast cereal.

Whole wheat pastry flour. Whole grain flour made from soft wheat. Used in baking items other than bread. Has a lower gluten content than regular flour, and is more nutritious.

Wild rice. The seed of an aquatic grass from a different botanical family from rice. It has a chewy, nutlike flavor. Use in place of rice. It has more protein and less starch than rice.

Yeast, rapid rise. This yeast is very porous so it hydrates quickly and easily. It cuts your baking time considerably because it doesn't need to be proofed; you can shape your dough right away.

APPENDIX 2

Equipment Glossary

B ELOW IS OUR alphabetical list of necessary or helpful tools for an ideal plant-based kitchen.

Blender Required for blending ingredients in many recipes in this book. Blenders produce a finer texture than food processors, because their blades move faster. The top-end blender is the Vita-Mix 5000, which can even cook soup as it blends! Less expensive brands are still quite good; we recommend Osterizer, Bosch, and Cuisinart.

Coffee grinder. A small, cheap electric coffee grinder works well for grinding seeds and nuts.

Colander. Plastic or steel, a colander, sometimes called a strainer, is used for draining and rinsing food. We recommend one large and one small.

Cookware. Pots, pans, and skillets coated with nonstick surfaces eliminate the need for added oil. Stainless steel, silicone-coated glass, iron, and porcelain also work well. Nonstick coated bakeware, such as loaf pans, cookie sheets, cake pans, and nonstick woks, are the most efficient and easiest to clean. When it comes to your budget, more expensive, quality cookware usually translates into longer lasting, better cooking results.

Cutting/Chopping boards. One large and one small are ideal. They can be wood, bamboo, or plastic, depending on your budget and taste. Always wash cutting boards thoroughly after each use. Flexible plastic chopping boards bend, making it easy to transfer chopped ingredients into a pot or bowl.

Food processor. Will save you endless time chopping, slicing, shredding, grinding, and pureeing. We recommend Bosch, Cuisinart, and Hamilton Beach brands.

Juicer. We recommend the Champion brand. While you don't need a juicer for our recipes, a good one can come in handy for making our Fresh Fruit Sorbet (page 248), as well as nut butters, and healthy, low-glycemic juices (try apple, kale, and carrot).

Knives. A good 7-inch chef's knife is essential. Keep it sharp. We also recommend an assortment of other sizes, particularly a 5-inch one with a serrated edge and a 3- or 4-inch paring knife. Henkels, Wusthof, and Cutco are all excellent mid-priced brands.

Measuring cups. Two sets are best: one for dry ingredients and one for wet. Dry measuring cups are usually solid plastic or metal, and allow for exact size measurement (you scrape the top and get an exact measurement). Liquid measuring cups are usually clear plastic or glass, and are marked with lines on the inside or outside showing you various quantities. Don't interchange these, as your measurements will be off.

Measuring spoons. Two sets are best, so you can measure wet and dry ingredients for the same recipe, without having to rinse between.

Pressure cooker. Good for cooking beans and stews in a hurry. The new types of pressure cookers are not as scary as they used to be, but *always follow the manufacturer's instructions* to avoid disaster. We recommend Kuhn-Rikon, Fagor, Wise, and Presto brands.

Slow cooker. A slow cooker, the "vegetarian's best friend," is ideal for cooking beans and stews. Choose a size that suits your cooking needs.

Steamer basket, collapsible. For steaming vegetables. Arrange the vegetables in the cradle of the steamer and place in a pot with 1 inch water in the bottom. You can save the liquid after steaming and use it for stock.

Stick (immersion) blender. This is a handheld blender with an electric motor on the top and rotating blade at the bottom. It can be placed directly into hot or cold soups, sauces, and drinks. We recommend KitchenAid, Cuisinart, and Braun brands.

Storage containers. Various sizes of glass or hard, clear plastic with plastic lids are recommended. The disposable kind you can buy at the supermarket are a good value and can be reused many times in the cupboard and refrigerator, but are not microwave-proof.

Toaster oven. Handy for toasting small quantities of nuts, drying bread crumbs, or roasting small servings of vegetables.

Waffle iron. Ideally, a regular (sometimes called American) waffle iron, as opposed to a Belgian waffle iron, will work best for the recipes in this book (regular waffles are thinner and denser, with smaller grooves). A round, 7-inch nonstick iron will work best. We especially like the Cuisinart, Hamilton Beach, and VillaWare brands.

Other Useful Items

In the long run, you can waste a huge amount of time and cause yourself aggravation or even injury if you don't have some basic tools of at least moderate quality. You could spend from $.99 up to $10 on each of these items. We'd recommend you stock your kitchen with the following items that are durable and fit into your price range.

- Brush, small, for basting
- Can opener, heavy duty (we recommend the old fashioned kind, not the flimsy tin kind)
- Garlic press
- Kitchen scissors
- Kitchen timer
- Ladle
- Microplane, for grating lemon and orange peel, and fresh ginger
- Mixing bowls, large, medium, and small
- Potato masher
- Scoop, ½ and ¼ cup, to form burgers and measure sorbets
- Sifter
- Spatula, (small) silicone or rubber, for scraping
- Spatula (wide paddle), silicone, for turning and flipping
- Tongs
- Vegetable peeler
- Whisks, various sizes
- Wooden spoons

Cooking Terms and Techniques

Al dente. An Italian phrase meaning "to the tooth," describing pasta or other food that is cooked only until it offers a slight resistance when bitten.

Blanch. To place food in cold water, bringing it to a boil for the time specified by the recipe, then draining well and refreshing in cold water to stop the cooking process. Works to loosen the skin of tomatoes for easier peeling, or to partially cook fresh green beans, peppers, or asparagus for use in a recipe.

Blend. To mix two or more ingredients together with a blender, beater, spoon, or electric mixer until well combined.

Boil. To heat a liquid until bubbles break the surface (212°F, 100°C at sea level and lower temperatures at higher altitudes). A "full rolling boil" is one that can't be dissipated by stirring.

Caramelize. To heat sugar or another food (e.g., onions) over low heat or in an oven until it develops a flavorful, golden-brown color. With sugar substitutes, this process might produce a chemical odor, but the final product and flavor will be fine.

Chiffonade. Long, thin ribbons of fresh greens (e.g., kale) or herbs made by rolling up the leaves and cutting crosswise.

Cream. To beat until light and fluffy.

Crudités (pronounced crew-di-TAYS). Raw vegetables, usually served with a dip or sauce.

Dice. To cut into small cubes.

Fold (in). To mix gently with a spoon.

Grill. To cook food on a heavy metal grate that is set over hot coals or other source of heat.

Julienne. To cut ingredients (e.g., vegetables) into thin, matchstick-size strips.

Marinate. To soak food (e.g., vegetables or tofu) in a seasoned liquid, so ingredients will absorb flavor and/or tenderize. Because most marinades contain an acid such as citrus juice, vinegar, or wine, marinating should be done in a glass, ceramic, or stainless steel container, and never in aluminum.

Mince. To finely dice.

Parboil. To partially cook in boiling water; the cooking is then completed by some other method.

Pulse. To turn blender/food processor on and off quickly so as not to overprocess ingredients (e.g., tomatoes).

Puree. To grind, blend, process, or mash food through a sieve until it forms a smooth, thick mixture, as for a soup.

Reduce. To decrease the volume of liquid via evaporation, by boiling rapidly in an uncovered pan. Reducing increases flavor and thickens consistency.

Sauté. To cook quickly in a small amount of oil over direct heat.

Shred. To cut food (e.g., soy cheese, carrots, or cabbage) into slivers or narrow strips, either by hand, hand-held grater, or food processor fitted with a shredding disk.

Sift. To remove lumps from a dry ingredient (e.g., flour) by passing it through a strainer or other fine mesh.

Simmer. To cook a liquid (e.g., soup) gently at a temperature that is low enough so that tiny bubbles just begin to break the surface.

Steam. To cook food (e.g., vegetables) on a rack or special steamer basket over boiling or simmering water in a covered skillet or saucepan.

Stir-fry. To cook small pieces of food quickly over very high heat while constantly and briskly stirring, until the food is hot and crisply tender. A wok or large skillet is usually used with this Asian cooking technique.

Whip. To beat ingredients (e.g., egg replacer) to incorporate air into them, thereby increasing their volume until they are the consistency described in the recipe.

Whisk. To beat or whip ingredients with a kitchen utensil that consists of a series of looped wires that form a three-dimensional teardrop shape.

Whiz. To rapidly blend wet or dry ingredients in a blender or food processor.

Zest. The colorful rind of citrus fruit (e.g., lemon, lime, or orange), containing aromatic oils that add flavor to food. When zesting, be careful to not include any of the white pith, as that adds a bitter taste.

Index

Page numbers in **bold** indicate tables.

About the Authors

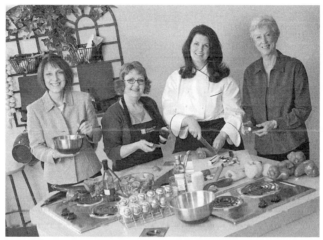

From left to right: Diana Fleming, Linda Kennedy, Linda Brinegar, and Bonnie House.

BONNIE HOUSE

In 1957, 19-year-old Bonnie married Dr. Franklin House, coauthor of *The 30-Day Diabetes Miracle* (Perigee, 2008). The biscuits she made during their honeymoon were suitable for hockey only—but of course Franklin ate them! Bonnie humbled herself and finally asked her mother, a vegetarian cooking master, to save her from kitchen fear and ignorance. In the '60s, Bonnie began testing, refining, and improvising with recipes from her mother and beyond. First she conquered whole wheat bread baking—she's made all her family's bread for 50 years. Mexican food, which Franklin craved since his childhood south of the border, was next. She's come a long way. In those days, Bonnie was a milk-, cheese-, and meat-lover: In the early '80s, she studied quiche-making from a French chef, and she and Franklin ran a cattle ranch, which provided home-grown beef. But Bonnie's father, the family patriarch, gave up all animal products for health reasons. That piqued her interest, because she'd suffered since girlhood from a painful joint condition no doctor could cure. So in the mid '80s, the Houses went on a quest to health centers across the country in search of the ideal diet for optimum health. That journey confirmed what they already suspected, that a total plant-based diet was ideal. Two weeks into her total plant-based diet, Bonnie was free of pain and pain medicine. That was 22 years ago, and she's adhered to a plant-based diet ever since. Back then, though, Bonnie's cooking style could best be characterized as trial-and-error. Many of the ingredients in plant-based cooking, even modern vegetarian staples like soymilk and tofu, were rare, and often had to be made from scratch. Bonnie persevered. With a degree in education, it was a natural for her to begin teaching two-week healthy-cooking classes to Franklin's patients who wanted freedom from chronic illness, and the skills and confidence to cook plant-based delights at home. Through this process she assembled hundreds of time-tested, mouthwatering plant-based recipes. She self-published several cookbooks, including *From Scratch* and *Oh Good, Soup*, which she also illustrated. In 2000 the Houses came to Lifestyle Center of America, where Franklin was president, and is now chairman of the board. Bonnie joined the circle of great chefs and teachers at LCA, and was a natural fit for the *30-Day Diabetes Miracle Cookbook*.

DIANA FLEMING, PH.D., LDN

IT'S IRONIC THAT most people with degrees in nutrition don't know how to cook—and many don't even manage to eat for optimal health. Not so with Diana. She has a passion for nutrition, and sticks to a healthy, totally plant-based diet. And she sure knows how to cook, too! As cofounder and comanager of Country Life Vegetarian Restaurants in New York and London, and later as vegetarian cooking consultant for the Wellesley College and Harvard University dining services, she's been a vanguard in plant-based nutrition, education, and food preparation for decades. Diana got her formal training at Tufts University, where she saw all four of her thesis papers published in the *American Journal of Clinical Nutrition*. She joined the staff at Lifestyle Center of America in 2002, and has served as Director of Nutritional Services since 2003. Diana specializes in nutrition education and counseling for people with diabetes. Her clients report her enthusiasm is infectious; her knowledge, invaluable; and her steadfastness necessary as a counterbalance to a culture of harmful excess. Diana's especially sensitive and empathetic when it comes to people with "food issues," because she's had a few herself: She's a former chocoholic and dessert junkie, whose own harrowing experience battling the temptation for unhealthy food has helped hundreds of clients, including coauthor Ian, overcome their own food demons.

LINDA BRINEGar

CREATING HEALTHY, GORGEOUS meals has been Linda B.'s passion for nearly 20 years, but actually, she's been cooking since she was five years old, as a student of two "fabulous grandma cooks." Her mother's a lifetime food service director, and Linda. B.'s honored to have followed in her footsteps. As food service director for a high school, college, convention center, and another health care facility, Linda B. has provided tens of thousands of people the gastronomic pleasure and health benefits of delicious, natural, health-restoring plant-based foods, prepared with loving care. She also ran her own healthy catering company, The Wooden Spoon, and has developed curricula and taught at cooking schools. Since 2004, she's directed Lifestyle Center of America's Windcrest Restaurant, where she supervises a staff of eleven. A self-taught chef, Linda B. still spends hours researching and perfecting her skills in the art and science of making healthy meals look and taste wonderful. Linda B. says all she does is take the brilliant, beautiful colors, flavors, and textures of wholesome, natural foods, and simply adds the finishing touch. But there's more to it than that. When a meal plan is so different from the Standard American Diet as ours is, people feel deprived unless the foods look and smell enticing—then a whole new world of culinary pleasure opens up. When Linda's not cooking, she's traveling the world as an avid birdwatcher.

LINDA KENNEDY

LINDA K. GOT a very early start on the culinary arts path in the fifth grade, when she and her brother began helping their hardworking mom cook the family suppers. She originally adopted a plant-based lifestyle 30 years ago for her asthmatic daughter's health. She credits the diet with saving her daughter and herself from respiratory symptoms and medication—and her husband, Ed, from heart disease. For 25 years, Linda K.'s been working in totally plant-based kitchens, where she's been a cook, a trainer, and a manager. Most recently she became a student when she attended an intensive summer training course at the Natural Gourmet Cookery school in New York. She was Food Service Director for the Oklahoma Academy boarding school before she co-coordinated the setup of Lifestyle of America's Windcrest Restaurant kitchen. In 1996, Linda K. became a sous chef, then managed the restaurant, and later assumed responsibility for directing the LCA Culinary Arts Program, where she's a popular teacher and nonstop inventor of new recipes. Linda K.'s specialty is converting "traditional" (read: high-fat, high-calorie, high-glycemic recipes laced with animal products) into more healthful, plant-based alternatives. Linda K. gets genuinely excited by the potential power of a plant-based lifestyle for diabetes, and always manages to incorporate the physical, mental, and spiritual benefits of healthy eating in all her interactions with her students. She's especially proud to teach people quick and easy recipes that taste great and restore health. Linda's also an accomplished artist and craftsman, but her greatest joy in life is being a grandma.

IAN BLAKE NEWMAN

IAN HAS TYPE-1 diabetes, and an insatiable appetite for delectable food and lots of it. A New York journalist, professor, college administrator, and motivational speaker, he is also the author and editor of *Managing the College Newsroom* (Associated Collegiate Press, 2003), and has twice been nominated for a Pushcart Prize. Ian first came to Lifestyle Center of America in 2005 in search of a miracle. His transformation was so radical that he continued a close association with its doctors and staff members, eventually coauthoring *The 30-Day Diabetes Miracle* (Perigee, 2008). A lifetime "semi-vegetarian," Ian honed his plant-based lifestyle and cooking skills during many visits to LCA, and credits it with literally saving his life. He shares Diana's love for chocolate, and also fears its dark side. Though Ian does most of the cooking at home, his partner, Dave, is a Culinary Institute of America–trained chef whose favorite cheesecake, Raspberry Swirl Cheesecake (page 268), now is low-fat, low-carb, and completely dairy-free.